Medical Information on the Internet

Dedication

To T. H. K.

For Churchill Livingstone:

Commissioning Editor: Michael Parkinson
Project Editor: Janice Urquhart
Project Controller: Nancy Arnott
Design Direction: Sarah Cape

Medical Information on the Internet

A Guide for Health Professionals

Robert Kiley BA(Hons) MSc ALA
Information Service Manager, Wellcome Trust, London

SECOND EDITION

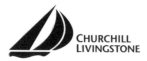
CHURCHILL
LIVINGSTONE

EDINBURGH   LONDON   NEW YORK   PHILADELPHIA   SYDNEY   TORONTO   1999

CHURCHILL LIVINGSTONE
An imprint of Harcourt Publishers Limited

First published 1996
Second edition 1999
Reprinted 2000
ISBN 0 443 06194 7

British Library Cataloguing in Publication Data
A catalogue record for this book is available from the
British Library.

Library of Congress Cataloging in Publication Data
A catalog record for this book is available from the
Library of Congress.

Medical knowledge is constantly changing. As new
information becomes available, changes in treatment,
procedures, equipment and the use of drugs become
necessary. The author and the publishers have, as far as
it is possible, taken care to ensure that the information
given in this text is accurate and up to date. However,
readers are strongly advised to confirm that the
information, especially with regard to drug usage,
complies with current legislation and standards of
practice.

The
publisher's
policy is to use
paper manufactured
from sustainable forests

Typeset by IMH(Cartrif) Loanhead, Scotland
Printed by Bell and Bain Ltd., Glasgow

Contents

Preface to the second edition

In the two and a half years that have elapsed since the first edition was published, the Internet has changed in many ways. Perhaps the most visible difference is the way the technologies of the Web and television have converged. WebTV is now a reality, and even if you still use an 'old fashioned' computer for accessing the Internet, an increasing number of Web sites are developing the idea of 'channels', that carry information aimed at a specific audience.

The same period has also witnessed an unprecedented growth in both the number of people who can access the Internet – from 30 million in March 1996 to 130 million in July 1998 – and the number of Web pages that can be accessed by any Internet user. A survey conducted by Digital Systems Research Center in March 1998 calculated that there were 275 million pages on the Web, and this was growing at a rate of 20 million pages a month.[1] Against this background, revising a book about the Internet is akin to hitting a moving target!

As with the first edition, I have concentrated on providing a *practical* guide to the Internet for health professionals. For example, rather than simply provide an exhaustive list of 'useful sites' I have focused instead on explaining how you can search the Internet and retrieve information specific to *your* needs. Similarly, when discussing e-mail, the emphasis is on practical considerations, such as how you can find someone's address and how you can use e-mail to send a fax to a colleague who is not yet connected to the Internet.

Recognising the growing concern about the quality of some of the health information that can be found on the Internet, this edition has a new chapter devoted to this topic. In addition to providing some examples of dubious health claims, I also highlight ways in which the quality of the information can be assessed, and describe a number of initiatives that are being developed to help manage this problem.

There is also a new chapter on consumer health information, which poses a number of 'patient questions' and looks at how these can be answered using resources that are freely available on the Internet. Throughout the analysis, emphasis is placed on the need to identify information that is both accurate and comprehensible to a lay audience.

All the other chapters have been extensively revised and rewritten. Chapter 2 includes updated information on getting connected to the Internet, along with details of service providers in both the UK and the US. Chapter 3 introduces a number of new search services, whilst a revised 'Top 10' is presented in Chapter 4.

The book's supporting Web pages[2] have also been redesigned. From these, you can access many of the resources discussed in this book and contact me with comments or suggestions for future editions.

Perhaps the only thing that has not changed since the first edition is my enthusiasm for the Internet and my belief that the information resources now available can help all health professionals deliver patient care more effectively.

Guildford, Surrey **Robert Kiley**
August 1998   rkiley@rkiley.demon.co.uk

REFERENCES

1 Digital Research
<URL: http://www.research.digital.com/SRC/ whatsnew/sem.html> [Accessed 1 August 1998]

2 Medical information on the Internet home page
<URL: http://www.hbuk.co.uk/kiley/>

Preface to the first edition

The Internet is everywhere. If you pick up a newspaper, you will find stories about it. On the radio and television you are as likely to hear e-mail addresses being cited as contact points, as telephone or fax numbers. Even advertisements, for items as diverse as beer and building societies, now include a reference to the product's presence on the World Wide Web.[1,2]

This interest in the Internet is not restricted to the popular media. Editors of medical journals accept articles about the Internet, welcome correspondence by e-mail; some actually publish via this medium. For example, the BMJ Classified Section, probably the most popular medical title in the UK, can now be accessed on the Internet.[3]

Being aware of the Internet, and being able to use it effectively, however, are two very different things. Indeed, in my role as a health sciences librarian I find that although the majority of health professionals have read about the Internet and are enthusiastic about its potential, few have any clear idea of how they can tap into this mass of information to find data relevant to their needs. Addressing this problem is one of the primary themes of this book.

In realising this objective, I have concentrated on providing practical illustrations of how the Internet can be of use to health professionals on a day-to-day basis. For example, although the section on Usenet Newsgroups explains what these are, the *focus* of the discussion looks at how a doctor/nurse/pharmacist etc. can identify newsgroups appropriate to their specific interests and issues such as how the 'news' can be filtered so that time is not wasted reading irrelevant mailings.

By concentrating on the practical aspects of how health professionals can make best use of the Internet, it is hoped that this book will be of use to both Internet novices and veterans.

One of the problems of writing about the Internet is the danger that it will be out of date before it is published. To minimise this risk, this book is complemented by a series of World Wide Web pages through which you can link to the key medical resources. You can also use these pages to mail me with comments and suggestions.[4]

The medical and health-related resources available on the Internet are vast. This book will introduce you to some of the key sites, but more importantly it will equip you with the necessary tools for you to undertake your own exploration.

Guildford, Surrey   **Robert Kiley**

REFERENCES

1 Guinness Home Page <URL: http://www.guinness.ie/>
2 Nationwide Building Society <URL: http://www.nationwide.co.uk/homepage/homepage.htm>
3 BMJ Classified <URL: http://www.bmj.com>

4 Churchill Livingstone Medical Information on the Internet <URL http://www.churchillmed.com/> (now harcourtbrace, see Preface to second edition)

Acknowledgements

I would like to thank the many people (most of whom I have never met) who took the time and trouble to respond to my requests for information. I would also like to express my thanks to the staff and users of the Wellcome Trust Information Service: a number of the information searches described here originated from reader requests.

I would especially like to thank my wife Genevieve for her continuing support and for the work she performed in proof reading the text.

August 1998   **Robert Kiley**

About the CD-ROM

Enclosed with this book you will find a free CD-ROM, containing the entire searchable text of the book, together with all the Internet screen grabs in colour.

This electronic file has been created as a 'pdf' (portable document format) file.

INSTALLATION INSTRUCTIONS

PC Single User, Local CD-ROM Installation

1. Exit all Windows programs including screen savers and virus software.
2. Insert the CD-ROM into the drive.

Windows 95 , 98 and NT 4.0

- From the desktop, double-click on **My Computer.**
- Double-click on the CD-ROM drive, which should display the name **Kiley** (*Drive Letter:*).
- Double-click on the **Setup** icon.

Setup

Windows 3.x

- From **Program Manager**, select **File**, **Run** and then type *d***:setup** (where *d* is the drive letter of your CD-ROM) and click **OK**.
- If you do not know the drive letter, select **Browse** and click on the down arrow in the **Drives** dialog box.
- Select your CD-ROM drive icon, click on setup.exe in the File Name dialog box, and select **OK**.
- Click on **OK** to begin the installation.

3. Click **Next** after reading the Welcome and Copyright Notice screens.
4. Select the default **Destination Folder** C:\Kiley or **Browse** for a different destination and click **Next**.
5. **CAREFULLY READ** the instructions regarding the options to install the entire contents of the CD-ROM to your hard disk or to perform a minimum installation. Select **OK**.
6. Select either **Leave data on the CD-ROM** or **Install data to hard disk** and click Next.
7. Choose the default Program Folder **Medical Information**, select an existing folder, or type a new folder name to be created and click **Next**.
8. Follow the instructions for installing Adobe Acrobat Reader.
9. Select **Yes** to restart the computer or Windows and complete the installation. Click **Finish**.

Macintosh Single User, Local CD-ROM Installation

1. Insert the CD-ROM into the drive.
3. Double-click on the **Double-click to Install** icon.
3. Click **Continue** on the startup screen.
4. Select **Agree** to begin installing.
5. Choose **Quit** to finish the installation.
6. Follow instructions for installing Adobe Acrobat Reader.
7. Select **Restart** to complete the installation.

UNINSTALL INSTRUCTIONS

PC

Windows 95, 98 and NT 4.0

1. From the desktop, click **Start** and scroll to **Programs** and choose **Medical Information.**
3. Select the **Uninstall** icon.
3. Choose **Yes** to completely remove **Medical Information** and all of its components.
4. After UnInstallShield has verified that all files and directories have been removed, select **OK**.

Windows 3.x

1. From Program Manager, open the **Medical Information** Program Group.
2. Double-click on the **Uninstall** icon.
3. Choose **Yes** to completely remove the product and all of its components.
4. After UnInstallShield has verified that all files and directories have been removed, select **OK**.

Macintosh

Locate the **Medical Information** folder and drag it to the **Trash**. Select **Empty Trash** from the Special menu.

You can also use the CD-ROM to connect directly to any of the Internet sites mentioned in the book, by double-clicking on the relevant URL (or Internet address). For this to work, you will need to be connected to the Internet and have a Web browser installed (see Ch. 2 for details).

Finally, you can access the home page for the book on the Harcourt Brace World Wide Web site. The address for the book's home page is:

http://www.hbuk.co.uk/kiley/

We hope you enjoy both the book and the accompanying CD-ROM.

1

Why use the Internet?

Box 1.1 Objectives of this book

- Explain, in a non-technical fashion, how you set about getting your computer connected to the Internet (Ch. 2).
- Demonstrate how you can find information on the Internet *specific* to your needs (Ch. 3).
- Alert you to some of the premier health and medical sites available on the Internet, and demonstrate how access to these can help you perform your day-to-day clinical work more effectively (Chs 4 and 5).
- Introduce you to some of the key communication services on the Internet and show how these can be used in a practical way (Ch. 6).
- Discuss the quality of the health information on the Internet, and provide some pointers to help you assess the information you retrieve (Ch. 7).
- Highlight a number of Web sites that provide answers to a range of typical consumer-health questions, and consider some of the ethical issues the Internet poses for health professionals (Ch. 8).
- Examine how the Internet is evolving and what impact this will have on the future delivery of health care (Ch. 9).

INTRODUCTION

Information is one commodity health professionals are not short of. A search of MEDLINE, for example, shows that in 1997 more than half a million new articles were indexed by this database. MEDLINE, however, is but one source of information. Guidelines, protocols and reports produced by government, professional associations and local groups all contribute to the information mountain, as do the numerous health stories and scares that appear in the popular press and consumer health magazines.

Consequently, with many health professionals already experiencing information overload – 'infoglut' – the prospect of accessing the Internet, where *more* health resources can be found, may appear somewhat daunting.[1,2,3] This feeling may be further exacerbated by thoughts that getting connected to the Internet, and subsequently finding relevant information, are both difficult, time-consuming tasks best left to computer whizz-kids. Indeed, a letter to the *BMJ* concluded that:

> *I have not counted the many hours spent in this exercise but I would advise only serious computer enthusiasts with plenty of spare time to access the Internet from home.*[4]

The purpose of this book is to allay these fears, and demonstrate how the Internet is becoming an indispensable tool for today's health professional.

To put the book in context, though, it is necessary to briefly examine the sources of medical information that can be accessed *without* connecting to the Internet.

MEDICAL INFORMATION – BEFORE THE INTERNET

Historically, medical information has always been well organised. Since 1879, with the launch of *Index Medicus*, health professionals have had access to bibliographic tools that can be used to identify published research. Over the years *Index Medicus* has been joined by other bibliographic indices, such as *Excerpta Medica* and *Psychological Abstracts*. The subsequent publication of these and other databases in an electronic format – typically on CD-ROM – has made the task of retrieving medical information a quick and relatively painless experience.

Finding research that has proved to be *effective* has also become easier in recent times, with the development of databases of systematic reviews such as the *Cochrane Database of Systematic Reviews* and the *NHS Centre for Reviews and Dissemination* (NHSCRD).

Consequently, a physician looking for some recent reviews and evidence on the effectiveness of hormone replacement therapy in preventing osteoporosis, for example, can, on visiting the local medical library, find highly relevant publications. Moreover, as the resources cited thus far are available *without* an Internet connection, is there a need for health professionals to get connected? Why this question can be answered with a resounding yes, is discussed below.

THE INTERNET FOR HEALTH PROFESSIONALS

Throughout this book you will find numerous examples that demonstrate why the Internet is so important. Box 1.2 summarises what the Internet provides for health professionals.

Perhaps the best way to demonstrate the potential of the Internet is through an example. Continuing with the HRT and osteoporosis subject search mentioned above, Box 1.3 shows just *some* of the sources that can currently be found on the Internet.

This single example demonstrates the range of material that is published on the Internet. It also highlights how the more established resources – MEDLINE and the Cochrane Library – have also migrated to the Internet, where they have been joined by numerous other resources which, prior to the development of the Internet, would have been unavailable.

USING THIS BOOK

A great deal of jargon is associated with the Internet. Whenever possible this will be kept to an absolute minimum, but when there is no alternative such terms will be underlined. On the Internet, underlining indicates a hypertext link to a related document. In this book the link is to the glossary, which can be found in Appendix E. To ensure that this convention does not cause unnecessary distraction, only the *first* occurrence of a glossary term in any chapter will be underlined.

Throughout the course of this book you will be introduced to a wide range of health

---

Box 1.2 Reasons for connecting to the Internet

- Current and up-to-date information. Even with today's modern publishing methods it can still take many weeks before research findings submitted for publication find their way into print. It takes even longer for the traditional bibliographic databases to index these items. The Internet, however, enables instant publishing and instant retrieval.

- Access to **both** traditional and new sources of information. If, for example, you were undertaking research into the aetiology of epiglottitis you could undertake a search of the MEDLINE database,[5] view a video on how you assess a child with this complaint,[6] and participate in an interactive self-assessment test on the subject.[7] It should also be noted that most of the information published on the Internet is **not** available through any other format.

- The functionality to access health resources throughout the world for the price of a local phone call. If you wanted to access a range of resources via your computer *before* the development of the Internet, it would have been necessary to dial a number of information providers, many of whom would not be accessible via a low-cost local telephone number.

- Access to all resources through one piece of software – the World Wide Web browser – thus minimising the time it takes to become 'Internet literate'.

- The opportunity to discuss medical issues with colleagues and experts from around the world through e-mail, discussion lists and newsgroups.

- The opportunity to pursue your research interests and continuing medical education studies from your own desktop, at a time that is convenient to you.

Box 1.3 HRT and osteoporosis – some relevant Internet resources

- A full-text consensus statement from the Society of Obstetricians and Gynaecologists of Canada, on osteoporosis and HRT[8] (Fig. 1.1).

- A MEDLINE subject search using the PubMED clinical query filter to limit the results to those articles that focus on therapy[9] (Fig. 1.2).

- Detailed abstracts from the Cochrane Database of Systematic Reviews.[10]

- A tutorial on postmenopausal osteoporosis, developed and published by staff at the University of Florida College of Medicine.[11]

- Information for consumers – treatment, support groups, etc. – from the National Osteoporosis Foundation[12] (Fig. 1.3).

- Clinical practice guidelines for the prevention and treatment of postmenopausal osteoporosis, developed by the American Association of Clinical Endocrinologists and the American College of Endocrinology.[13]

- A full-text article from the evidence-based medicine journal, *Bandolier*, on the effectiveness of HRT for managing osteoporosis.[14]

- Gross and microscopic images of the vertebral bone with osteoporosis[15] (Fig. 1.4).

- A risk assessment score sheet to determine whether you are at risk of developing osteoporosis.[16]

---

resources available on the Internet. Some will be interactive, such as the Interactive Patient, where you 'interview' the client in an attempt to diagnose the illness. Some will use multimedia features such as audio and video. Others will simply be text. Whatever the medium, emphasis will be placed on how you can find appropriate information quickly and efficiently.

It should also be noted that the overwhelming majority of Internet resources are available free of charge. Although some sites, such as Medical Matrix and Medscape, for example,

may insist that you complete an online registration form before an 'access ID' is granted, there are no charges associated with registration. Consequently, unless *explicitly* stated, all the Internet sites listed in this book are available to any Internet user, free of charge. The only costs you will incur are those levied by your telecommunications and Internet providers.

To help you get a feel of what the Internet looks like, many of the examples cited here will be supported with screen shots. When no screen shot is provided, the full Internet address, known as the uniform resource locator (URL), will be cited. For example, the URL of the American Medical Association is:

http://www.ama-assn.org/

Once your Internet connection is in place (Ch. 2) you can jump directly to any cited

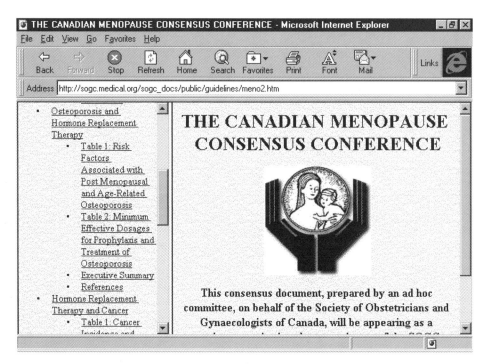

Fig. 1.1 Society of Obstetricians and Gynaecologists of Canada

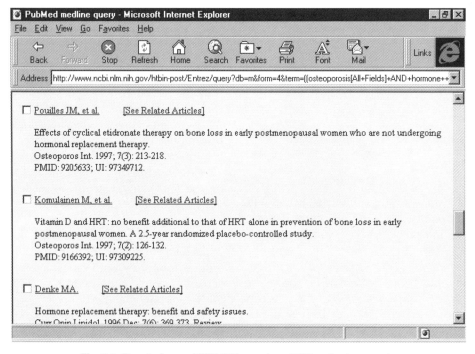

Fig. 1.2 Results from a MEDLINE search on HRT and osteoporosis

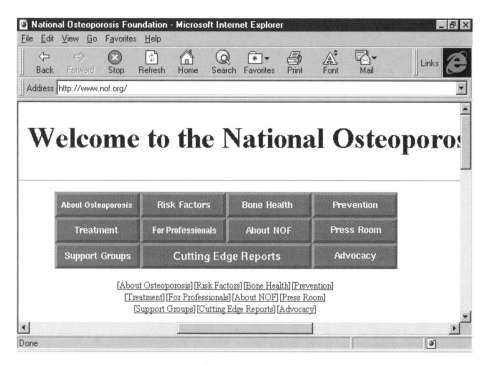

Fig. 1.3 Information for consumers from the National Osteoporosis Foundation

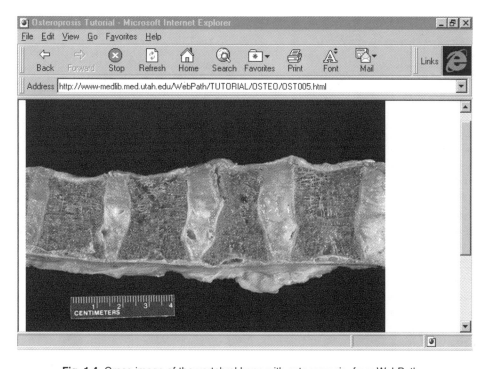

Fig. 1.4 Gross image of the vertebral bone with osteoporosis, from WebPath

resource through your World Wide Web browser. Both Netscape and the Internet Explorer – the two most popular Web browsers – have a 'location' window where you can input the URL *exactly* as it is shown. As many of the computers that make up the Internet are UNIX-based the case of the address is significant. In the example given below, merely entering BANDOLIER in capital letters will cause your Web browser to report that the file 'cannot be found'.

http://www.jr2.ox.ac.uk/bandolier/ ✔

http://www.jr2.ox.ac.uk/BANDOLIER/ ✗

Further details of how to use both Netscape and the Internet Explorer can be found in Appendix B.

However, before you can begin to search for information on the Internet, or even visit the URL cited above, you need to get your computer hooked up. Chapter 2 looks at how this can be achieved and at what cost.

REFERENCES

1 Laskin DM 1994 Dealing with information overload [editorial]. Journal of Oral and Maxillofacial Surgery 52(7):661
2 Hendee WR 1991 Information overload and management in radiology. AJR American Journal of Roentgenology 156(6):1283–1285
3 Faber RG 1993 Information overload [letter]. BMJ 307(6900):383
4 David T. 1996 Accessing the Internet is far from easy [letter]. BMJ 312(7022):55
5 PubMed Medline <URL: http://ncbi.nlm.nig.gov/ PubMed> [Accessed 19 June 1998]
6 Virtual Hospital <URL: http:// vh.radiology.uiowa.edu/Providers/Textbooks/ ElectricAirway/Video/epibronc.mov> [Accessed 19 June 1998]
7 Virtual Hospital <URL: http:// vh.radiology.uiowa.edu/Providers/Textbooks/ ElectricAirway/Text/Epiglottitis.html> [Accessed 19 June 1998]
8 Society of Obstetricians and Gynaecologists of Canada <URL: http://sogc.medical.org/sogc_docs/ public/guidelines/meno2.htm> [Accessed 19 June 1998]
9 PubMed Medline – Clinical Query Filter <URL: http://www.ncbi.nlm.nih.gov/PubMed/ clinical.html> [Accessed 19 June 1998]
10 Cochrane Database of Systematic Reviews <URL: http://www.cochrane.co.uk/abstracts/ ab000952.htm> [Accessed 19 June 1998]
11 University of Florida College of Medicine <URL: http://www.medinfo.ufl.edu/cme/osteo/ osteo1.html> [Accessed 19 June 1998]
12 National Osteoporosis Foundation <URL: http:// www.nof.org/> [Accessed 19 June 1998]
13 AACE <URL: http://www.aace.com/clin/guides/ osteoporosis.html> [Accessed 19 June 1998]
14 Bandolier <URL: http://www.jr2.ox.ac.uk/Bandolier/ band3/b3-4.html> [Accessed 19 June 1998]
15 WebPath <URL: http://www-medlib.med.utah.edu/ WebPath/TUTORIAL/OSTEO/OSTEOPOR.html> [Accessed 19 June 1998]
16 The Osteoporosis Center <URL: http://www.sonnet.com/usr/imaging/ SCORE.html> [Accessed 16 June 1998]

2

Getting wired

Box 2.1 Chapter objectives

- Explain what the Internet is.

- Introduce some of the key Internet services, such as e-mail and the World Wide Web.

- Provide a checklist of items required for Internet access.

- Detail the services and prices of the leading Internet service providers in the UK and the US.

- Provide typical costing for Internet connectivity.

INTRODUCTION

Having seen that the Internet can provide you with relevant, timely and unique information resources, it is necessary to set about the task of getting connected. Before doing this, however, it is important to have some understanding of what the Internet actually is.

What is the Internet?

Put simply, the Internet is just a network of computer networks that spans the globe. In terms of size, a survey conducted in January 1998 calculated that around 30 million computers are connected to Internet, providing connectivity in over 190 countries.[1]

What makes the Internet so remarkable is the fact that all these computers, on all these separate networks, can all communicate with each other. This situation has been made possible by the fact that they all speak the same language. For the more technically minded, all computers connected to the Internet use the same protocols, namely TCP/IP (transmission control protocol/internet protocol).

This agreed protocol also means that the Internet is not platform dependent. Although it may be slightly more complicated to get an Amiga or Atari computer connected – in the sense that there is less Internet software available for such platforms – once a version of TCP/IP has been installed these computers will be able to carry out the same Internet functions as an Apple Macintosh, an IBM-compatible computer, or indeed a UNIX-based system.

For the beginner, one of the key things to remember is that there is no central 'Internet computer'. For example, when you require a document published by the National Institutes of Health you obtain it directly from a computer (known as a server) located within the NIH. Similarly, to see this week's edition of the *Weekly Epidemiological Report*, produced by the World Health Organization, the WHO server in Geneva is accessed.

If, however, you are going to access the Internet through the telephone network, the prospect of reading and fetching files from around the world raises the spectre of high telephone bills. Although access costs are discussed more fully below, it should be stressed that once you connect to your Internet provider – ideally via a local telephone number – there are no further costs relating to distance. In other words, for a UK user it costs no more to fetch a file from a server in Australia than it does to obtain it from a server in London. And, strange as it may seem, if the Australian server is quiet (perhaps you are accessing it when local users are asleep) and the London server busy, you may actually get information delivered more quickly – and therefore more cheaply – from the site on the other side of the world.

History of the Internet

Originally devised in the 1960s as a project to ensure that military personnel could continue to communicate with each other in the event of war, the Internet has evolved into a network that interconnects government and education, and more recently business and commerce.

To meet the original objective the network was built on the premise that if one part of it failed – in Cold War terms a city might be knocked out by a nuclear strike – then the message (or file) would be routed via another part. This rerouting would continue until the message reached the intended recipient.

Although today networks are more likely to be brought down by workmen digging up cables, the same architecture is still in place. If you look at the top part – known as the header – of any e-mail message you will see the route the mail has taken. Every server that forwards the mail 'stamps' it with its name, and the date and time.

The explosion of interest in the Internet is, however, a relatively recent phenomenon. In 1981, the Internet Society counted 500 host computers on the Internet. Ten years later this figure had increased to 100 000. By 1998 this number had soared to more than 30 million.[2,3]

This massive upturn in the popularity of the Internet was bought about by the development of the World Wide Web, and more specifically the release, in December 1993, of Mosaic, the first graphical World Wide Web browser.

Moreover, this explosion of interest in, and development of, the Internet shows no sign of abating. A survey conducted by the Digital Systems Research Center in March 1998 calculated that there were at least 275 million distinct, static pages on the World Wide Web. More spectacularly, this survey showed that the Web had doubled in size in less than 9 months and is currently growing at about 20 million pages per month.[4]

KEY INTERNET SERVICES

Although the terms Internet and World Wide Web tend to be used synonymously, the Web is just one of a number of services carried by the Internet. This section will introduce you to some of the most important – and useful – Internet services. However, this is not an exhaustive list. Facilities such as 'Ping' – through which you can check whether another computer on the network is available – or the more mysterious-sounding 'finger', will not be discussed. If you require information on these, and other advanced Internet tools, see the *Internet Starter Kit for Windows* by Adam Engst, available in full-text at:

**http://www.mcp.com/resources/
 geninternet/iskm/iskw2/toc.htm**

E-mail – electronic mail

The desire to communicate electronically with colleagues and friends is still the principal reason why people seek Internet connectivity. In its simplest form e-mail can be used to send messages consisting of nothing other than text from one location to another. Beyond this it can be used to send binary files, such as word-processed documents, or act as an information retrieval tool.[5]

The popularity of e-mail can be put down to the following factors: it is cheap, easy to use, quick, and very efficient. Chapter 6 amplifies these points, and demonstrates why it has become such an indispensable tool for all Internet users.

World Wide Web – WWW

The development of the World Wide Web has provided the Internet with a multimedia interface. Using a mark-up language known as HTML, Web documents (called pages) can include text, graphics, moving images and sound. To 'read' a Web page you need a Web browser, such as the Netscape Navigator or the Microsoft Internet Explorer (see Appendix B for details of how to use Netscape and Internet Explorer).

The undoubted strength of the Web is the way related documents are seamlessly linked. As you scroll through a Web page various words and phrases are highlighted or underlined, indicating that these are hypertext links (Fig. 2.1). Mouse-clicking on one of these links sends a command to your Web browser to access this related resource. The page that is subsequently displayed may reside within the same file as the original document, in a different file on the same server, or in a different file on a different server anywhere in the world.

Because the Web is recognised as the 'killer application', relatively little attention is now

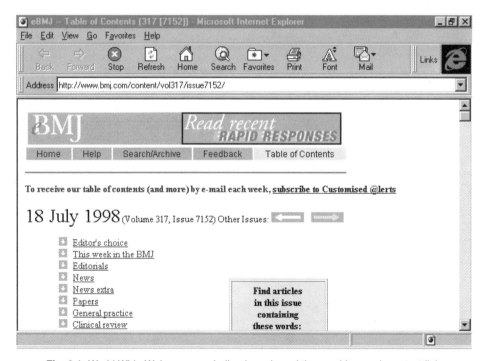

Fig. 2.1 World Wide Web page: underlined words and the graphics are hypertext links

paid to its immediate predecessor, Gopher. Gophers provided the first menu-driven, text-based interface to the Internet. However, as Gopher resources can be accessed through your Web browser they will not be dealt with separately in this book.

File transfer protocol

File transfer protocol (FTP) is the set of rules that govern how files on the Internet are moved from one location to another. Although in practice most FTP'ing is now done through the Web browser, FTP client software is necessary if you wish to upload files to your Web site. For further information about FTP see 'Finding and FTP'ing software' below.

Telnet

Telnet is a service that enables you to connect to remote computers on the Internet and use them in the same way as you would if you were sitting in front of them. Unlike the Web, however, Telnet does not support a graphical interface (Fig. 2.2). The task of having to

remember obscure keystroke commands, such as hitting the Ctrl and X keys simultaneously to end a Telnet session, can be a difficult and frustrating experience after the elegance and simplicity of the Web.

Because of these perceived difficulties, owners of Telnet sites are beginning to make their services available via the Web. However, until this process is complete, if you wish to access resources such as the catalogue of the Bodleian Library, Oxford,[6] then Telnet is your only option.

Usenet News

Usenet News – or network news as it is sometimes called – is the Internet equivalent of a bulletin board. Through this Internet service it is possible to engage in a subject-specific *group* discussion with other Internet users. Many of these groups are highly specialised, as is testified by the fact that there are approximately 30 000 newsgroups. Chapter 6 will look in more detail at this subject, and highlight those newsgroups that will be of most interest to health professionals.

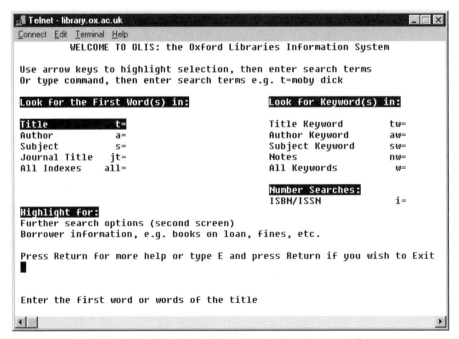

Fig. 2.2 Searching the Bodleian Library book catalogue via Telnet

GETTING CONNECTED

The purpose of this section is to give practical advice on how you can get your computer connected to the Internet. In doing this it will be assumed that the connection will be made via a dial-up commercial Internet provider. If you already have access to the Internet via JANET, NHSnet or some other institutional network, and you do not wish to have a connection at home, some of the following discussion may not be relevant.

Perhaps the first thing to state is that getting connected to the Internet is *not* difficult. Although a glance through the books in any computer bookstore may cause you to doubt this assertion, for most users it is no more complicated than installing any other piece of software on your computer. Most Internet service providers supply their subscribers with a suite of software, all of which can be installed and configured using clear and unambiguous 'wizards'. Box 2.2 identifies the sum total of items needed for Internet connectivity. Further details of these components are discussed below.

The computer

It is possible to connect almost any computer, with any specification, to the Internet. However, if you want to enjoy the benefits of a graphical environment (Windows or Macintosh), then the minimum *acceptable* configuration is a computer with a 486 processor that has at least 4 MB of RAM (Random Access Memory). In practice, though, a Pentium PC running Windows95 – a 32-bit operating system – with 16 or 32 MB of RAM will make the 'Internet experience' more enjoyable. With this type of specification, true multitasking – receiving mail in one window while browsing the Web in another – can be enjoyed.

Modem or terminal adapter?

Modems and terminal adapters (TAs) are the clever bits of equipment (hardware) that connect a computer to a data transmission line; in

---

> **Box 2.2** Necessary components for Internet connectivity
>
> - A computer
> - A modem or terminal adapter
> - A telephone or ISDN line
> - An account with an Internet provider
> - Internet communication and application software.

the case of connecting to the Internet this will be the telephone or the ISDN line.

Your decision on whether to purchase a modem or a TA will depend on the speed with which you want to access the Internet, how much money you want to spend, and whether your Internet service provider (see below) can support ISDN access. Whichever method you opt for it is a good idea to ask your Internet provider to recommend a modem or TA. If you do experience problems establishing a connection, the fewer variables in the equation the better: buying a modem or TA that your provider knows has not caused any problems to other users, removes one such variable.

Table 2.1 compares the relative merits of the modem with the terminal adapter.

Choosing an Internet provider

An Internet provider is someone who has a permanent connection to the Internet and who, for a fee, will let you use this route. Once connected to your provider via the telephone line, you are effectively connected to the Internet. You will have your own unique Internet address, be able to transfer files directly to your hard disk, and access such facilities as the World Wide Web, Usenet News and e-mail. When you have finished browsing the Web, or sending your mail, you log off. As your provider remains connected all the time any mail sent to you when you are not connected is held by them and delivered to you when you next log on.

Choosing an Internet provider, however, is not straightforward. As I write, in April 1998, there are more than 200 companies in the UK

Table 2.1 Modem or terminal adapter?

	Modem	Terminal adapter (TA)
Fastest access speed	56 Kbps. (V90 ITU standard.) Under this standard, modems are capable of receiving data at 56 Kbps and sending data at 33.6 Kbps	64 Kbps (or 128 Kbps if both data channels are used).
Data line	Telephone line	ISDN line
Hardware cost	Approx. £150.00	Approx. £250.00
Advantages	• No need for a separate data line • If you travel with your computer you are more likely to find a telephone line to plug a modem into than an ISDN line to accommodate your TA	• High access speeds and fast log-ons can be enjoyed • Calls charged at same price as ordinary phone calls • Digital line. Little or no data corruption • ISDN supports 'Multi-subscriber number-ing'. This allows you to plug a fax machine – with its own unique number – into the TA, thus negating the need for a separate line
Disadvantages	• The analogue telephone line – devised in the 19th century – is always going to be subject to line noise and data corruption	• Installation of ISDN line and rental charges are significantly higher than that charged for a telephone line

offering Internet connectivity. To help select the provider that can best address your needs, consider first what level of service you require:

- **Level 1 – E-mail only.** This may appeal to users who perhaps have full Internet access at their place of work – and thus can use services such as the WWW and FTP – but require a personal, private mail account at home. Table 2.2 gives details of two providers (one in the UK and one in the US) who offer this service.
- **Level 2 – Full Internet access.** With this level of service users get an e-mail account plus full access to all Internet services, such as WWW, Usenet, Newsgroups and FTP. Most providers offering this service also give subscribers Web space, thus enabling them to create their own pages on the WWW. Tables 2.3 and 2.4 provide details of the biggest providers – in terms of subscribers – operating in the UK and the US, who offer this service.
- **Level 3 – Full Internet access *plus* exclusive provider content.** With this option

subscribers enjoy full Internet access, plus services and content that are provider-specific. Details of providers offering this service are given in Table 2.5.

Other things to consider include the level of support on offer – is it available in the evening and weekends, and can you get through to it – and whether or not the provider will supply you with a suite of Internet-ready software that can be installed with ease? Also, try asking friends and colleagues to learn first-hand how the claims made by Internet providers match up in practice.

For information on other Internet service providers visit your local newsagent and scan through some of the current Internet magazines (Appendix A). Once you have access to the Internet, a complete listing of UK and US providers and the services they offer can be found at:

http://www.limitless.co.uk/inetuk (for UK providers) and

http://www.boardwatch.com (for US providers).

Table 2.2 E-mail access only

Provider	Joining fee	Monthly fee	Local-call access?	Maximum connect speed
CableNet (UK)	£15.00	£2.50	Yes	56 Kbps
Comments	Unlimited number of e-mail addresses for each account			
Contact	Phone: UK 01424 830700			
	http://www.cablenet.net			
Juno (US)	Free	Free	400 PoPs in the US	33.6 Kbps
Comments	The service is funded by advertising. Every mail message you receive is accompanied by 'banner advertisements'. If you need technical support this is charged at $1.95 per minute (Fig. 2.3)			
Contact	Phone: US 900 555-JUNO			
	http://www.juno.com			

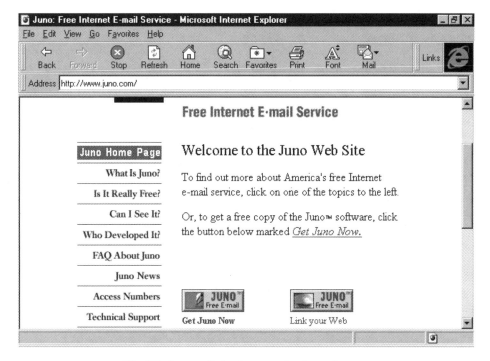

Fig. 2.3 Juno – offering free e-mail-only service

Table 2.3 Full Internet access (UK)

Provider	Joining fee	Monthly fee	Local-call access?	Subscribers	Maximum connect speed
Demon Internet (UK)	£12.50	£10.00	Yes	140 000	56 Kbps and ISDN
Comments	UK's largest independent Internet service provider, Demon Internet pioneered the 'tenner-a-month' access account. Demon owns its own 45 <u>Mbps</u> connection to the US. Backbone in UK runs at 155 Mbps and to the rest of Europe at 30 Mbps (Fig. 2.4)				
Contact	Phone: UK 0181 371 1000				
	http://www.demon.net				
BT Internet (UK)	Free	£11.75	Yes	100 000	56 Kbps and ISDN
Comments	Despite being the key player in the UK telecommunications industry, BT was relatively slow in offering Internet access. It is now a major player, offering services to home, school and business users. Members receive 5 MB Web space to create their own home pages and access to 24 hour support				
Contact	Phone: UK 0800 515585				
	http://www.bt.com/internet/index.htm				

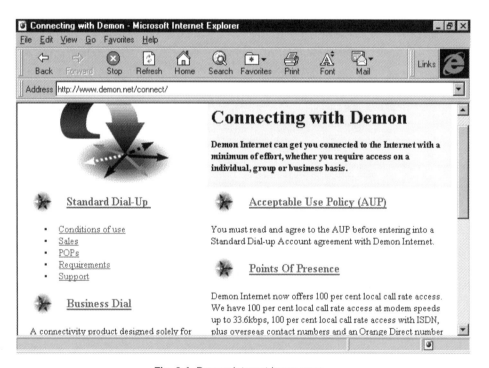

Fig. 2.4 Demon Internet home page

Table 2.4 Full Internet access (US)

Provider	Joining fee	Monthly fee	Local-call access?	Subscribers	Maximum connect speed
AT&T WorldNet (US)	Free	$19.95 for 150 hours; additional hours $0.99	Yes – access via 130 area codes	850 000	56 Kbps
Comments	A survey in *PC Magazine* commented that WorldNet's 'automated installation script [made it] one of the fastest and easiest services to set up. Within 15 minutes we were surfing the Web, sending e-mail, and accessing newsgroups'.[7] Access to the 56 Kbps service however, is only available in 11 cities; the remaining PoPs offer connectivity at 28.8 Kbps (Fig. 2.5).				
Contact	Phone: US 800 967 4906 **http://www.att.net**				
NetCom (US)	Free	$19.95, for access at 28.8 Kbps	Yes – access via 129 area codes	580 000	28.8 Kbps; 56 Kbps and ISDN
Comments	With its own fibreoptic network, Netcom offers fast and easy Internet access throughout the United States. In addition to the usual Internet services, subscribers also receive a copy of McAfee Webscan, which gives virus protection when sharing and exchanging files. For an additional fee subscribers can take advantage of the 'Global Roaming' service, which allows users to access the service – at local call rate – in UK and Canada.				
Contact	Phone: US 800 638 2661 **http://www.netcom.com**				

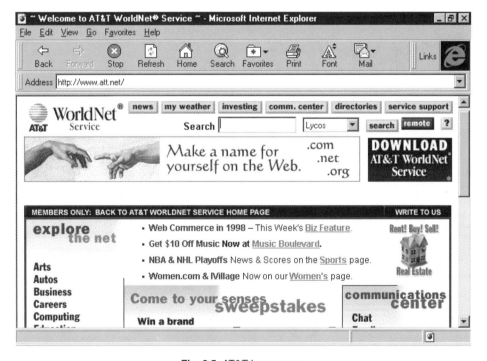

Fig. 2.5 AT&T home page

Table 2.5 Full Internet access and provider content (UK and US)

Provider	Joining fee	Monthly fee	Local-call access?	Subscribers	Maximum connect speed
AOL	Free	£16.95 / $21.95	Yes (UK). Access via 147 US area codes	11 million	33.6 Kbps
Comments	Members-only AOL channels cover topics such as news, sport, weather and learning. Users who do not require unlimited access to the Internet can opt for a £4.95 ($9.95) monthly subscription, which allows 3 free hours online, plus unlimited use of member services. Additional online time charged at £2.35 ($2.95) per hour (Fig. 2.6)				
Contact	Phone contacts 0800 376 5432 (UK); 800 827 6364 (US)				
	Address: **http://www.aol.com**				
	UK address: **http://www.aol.co.uk**				
CompuServe	Free	£6.50 / $9.95 (Limited to 5 hours' access time per month)	Yes (UK). Access via 152 US area codes	5.2 million	56 Kbps and ISDN
Comments	CompuServe has points of presence (PoPs) in more than 185 countries, thus ensuring that if you do a lot of international travelling and wish to use your computer notebook to send mail and surf the Web, it is likely there will be a local CompuServe number you can dial into (Fig. 2.7)				
	Members-only services include a number of special interest communities – including medical forums and a health database – plus access to Hutchinson Encyclopaedia, Electronic Yellow Pages and prices and reports from the London stock market. Online time in excess of the 5 free hours is charged at £1.95 ($2.95) per hour.				
Contact	Phone contacts: 0990 000 400 (UK); 800 848 8990 (US)				
	Address: **http://www.compuserve.com/**				
	UK address: **http://www.compuserve.co.uk**				
MSN	Free	£14.95 / $19.95	Yes (UK). Access via 149 US area codes	Not available	56 Kbps + ISDN
Comment	Access to MSN network available in the UK, US, Canada, Australia, France, Japan and Germany. Members-only content includes 40 international forums, Microsoft Expedia Travel Service, Encarta Encyclopaedia, and various financial services.				
Contact	Phone contacts: 0870 601 1000 (UK); 800 373 3676 (US)				
	Address: **http://www.msn.com/**				
	UK address: **http://www.uk.msn.com/**				

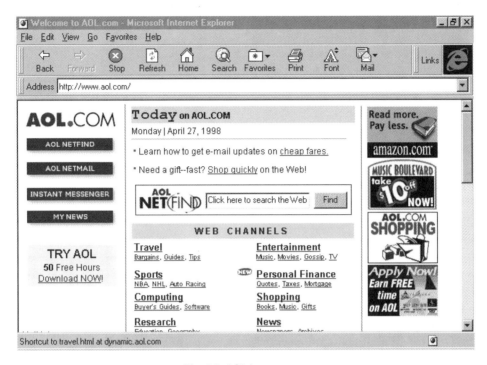

Fig. 2.6 AOL home page

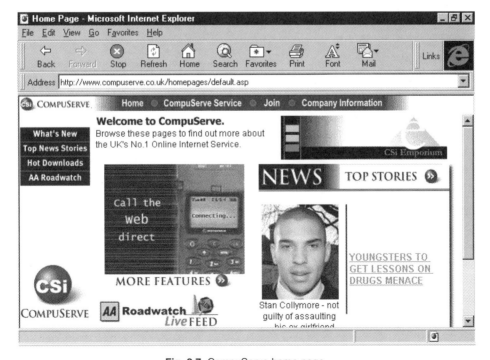

Fig. 2.7 CompuServe home page

INTERNET COMMUNICATION AND APPLICATION SOFTWARE

To be able to connect to the Internet, through your provider, you must use communications software that supports the Internet protocol TCP/IP. Programs such as *Windows Terminal* or *HyperTerminal* do **not** support this protocol and therefore cannot be used.

In addition to acquiring TCP/IP, you will also need a copy of either SLIP or PPP software. These are 'drivers' that enable TCP/IP to work over serial lines, such as the telephone network. As your Internet provider will supply you with copies of the required software and drivers, plus additional software to help you install and configure them, further explanation of TCP/IP, SLIP and PPP is unnecessary. They are mentioned here simply to reinforce the fact that you need these additional items *before* you can connect to the Internet. Appendix D provides an example of how TCP/IP can be configured under the Windows95 operating system.

The final thing you will need before you can start exploring the wonders of the Internet is some application software. For example, to send and receive e-mail you need an e-mail program; to view pages on the World Wide Web you need a Web browser.

Most applications you use on the Internet are based on the client–server model. In simple terms this means that you have a copy of the software on your computer (the client) that processes requests to other computers (servers) on the Internet. For the Internet user the advantages of this model are twofold: first, all the processing power of your computer can be harnessed and exploited, and secondly, you get to use the Internet via a graphical interface.

As mentioned earlier, your Internet provider should supply you with a suite of applications to get you started. However, as soon as you wish to add to or change the software you use, then the resources of the Internet are at your fingertips. One of the things you will not find in short supply on the Internet is software!

To move files (in this case software) from a server on the Internet to your computer you use the Internet protocol FTP.

Finding and FTP'ing software

The techniques discussed in Chapter 3 for finding medical information can also be used to identify where a particular computer program can be found on the Internet. For example, to acquire a new e-mail client you can visit the Yahoo! index[8] and follow the hypertext links from 'Computers and Internet' to 'Software' and Networking', and through to 'Electronic-Mail'. At this juncture you will find yourself presented with a choice of around 30 different e-mail programs.

Once you have identified which piece of software you require it can be FTP'd to your computer by simply mouse-clicking on the file name. The Web browser will immediately realise that the file cannot be viewed and suggest that it should be saved to disk. Depending on which browser you are running, you may see a 'saving' dialogue box that indicates how much of the file has been transferred, and approximately how long it will take to complete this task (Fig. 2.8).

An alternative approach to finding software is to visit a suitably large archive and browse. One of the biggest repositories of Internet software is held at TUCOWS (The Ultimate Collection of Winsock Software). Here, software is arranged by platform – Windows95, Macintosh, NT4.0 etc. – and then by application type. Once you have selected your area of interest a list of files is displayed, complete with annotations that tell you when the software was written, how big it is and what licence restrictions apply (Figs 2.9, 2.10).

To use the TUCOWS service, point your browser at: **http://www.tucows.com** This site is mirrored in many locations throughout the world, so for faster downloads you are encouraged to use your 'local' server.

Installing FTP'd software

To speed up data transfer most software applications are delivered to your computer in a compressed format. This will take the form of either a self-extracting archive or a packed file. In the former case you simply need to run the program to create all the necessary files and

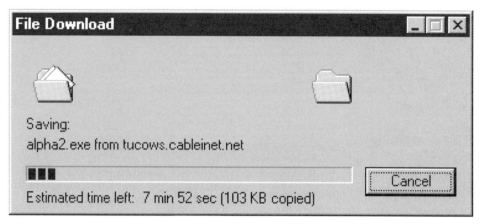

Fig. 2.8 Saving a file to disk

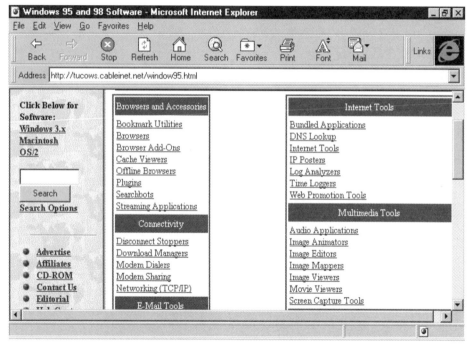

Fig. 2.9 The TUCOWS archive

directories. If it has been packed you will need to unpack it. Decompression utilities can be found at the TUCOWS site. Once unpacked, instructions on how to install the software will be found in a 'readme' file.

Shareware and Freeware

Newcomers to the Internet are often amazed at how easy it is to FTP software, and to do so without having to quote any credit card details. Most software on the Internet is classified as shareware, which normally means that you are entitled to use it and evaluate it for a period of around 30 days. If you wish to continue using the software after this time you are obliged to register your copy, and pay a fairly nominal licence fee.

Registration not only legitimises your use of the software, but may also entitle you to

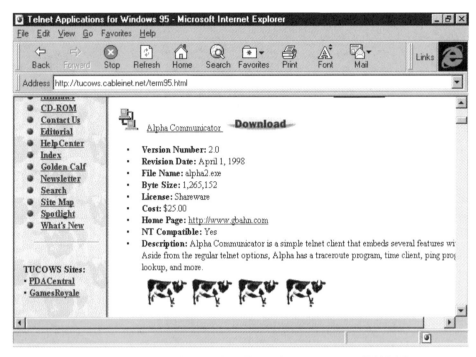

Fig. 2.10 Descriptions of some of the Telnet clients available at TUCOWS

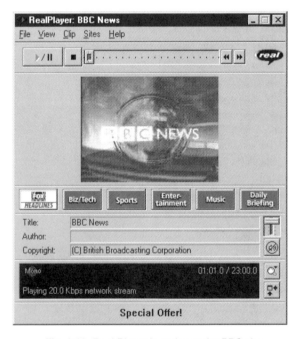

Fig. 2.11 Real Player in action at the BBC site

Table 2.6 Useful helper applications

Name	Purpose, cost and availability
Telnet	To enable you to run Telnet sessions. A choice of Telnet clients can be found at the TUCOWS site
	Available from: **http://www.tucows.com/**
Adobe Acrobat	A growing number of Web sites contain files in a 'pdf' format. Documents published in this way appear in precisely the same way as in the original paper version. Fonts, page layout, pagination etc. are all retained. Further, a pdf file can *only* be viewed: it cannot be edited
	Software cost: Free
	Available from: **http://www.adobe.com**
Real Player	Some Web sites – such as the BBC – carry live broadcasts on the Internet. To hear and see these a 'Real Player' is required (Fig. 2.11)
	Software cost: Free
	Available from: **http://www.realaudio.com**
Shockwave	To view Web-based animations written with Macromedia Director software, the Shockwave plug-in is required
	Software cost: Free
	Available from: **http://www.macromedia.com/**
QuickTime	A number of Web sites have movie clips stored as Quicktime files. To view these a Quicktime player is required
	Software cost: Free
	Available from: **http://www.apple.com/quicktime**

some additional documentation or e-mail support.

Other useful utilities

Your Web browser can be called upon to carry out many more functions than simply displaying World Wide Web pages. It can FTP as competently as a specific FTP program. It can also be used to send, and, if your Internet provider has a POP3 mail server, receive e-mail. It can also display bitmap (bmp) and JPEG images and play audio clips.

Nevertheless there will still be occasions when you will need an additional piece of software – typically referred to as helper applications – before you can access the information you have found. Table 2.6 details some of the more useful helper applications you may wish to FTP and install.

One other piece of software worth acquiring is a virus checker. Although the hype about viruses on the Internet has been overplayed, they do exist and should be taken seri-

ously. Viruses such as the 'winword.concept' – which hides itself as a macro in a Microsoft Word template document – demonstrate the 'skill' and ingenuity of the people who create them. Chapter 6 provides more information about e-mail viruses.

To negate this threat, all Internet users should invest in antivirus software *and* keep it updated. Before purchasing this, however, check with the supplier that the software can check *compressed* files for viruses. If a virus is within a piece of software, simply 'unpacking' it may infect your computer.

COSTS

Perhaps the most surprising thing about the Internet is how little it all costs. Leaving aside telephone charges for the moment, the cost of one year's access to the Internet is likely to be around £120.00. When you consider that a personal subscription to a journal such as the *Lancet* is a similar sum, you begin to appreciate what good value the Internet is.[9] Table 2.7

Table 2.7 Getting connected: costs

Description	Average cost
Modem (one-off cost)	£150.00
Internet provider membership fee (one-off cost)	£12.00
Annual subscription to your Internet provider	£120.00
Total cost for year 1 (excluding VAT)	£282.00

details all the initial charges you are likely to incur.

Although telephone costs are the great variable in the cost equation, they are the one feature that you have total control of. To help keep them to an affordable level, I suggest you adhere to the points in Box 2.3.

CONCLUSION

This chapter has demonstrated that connecting your computer to the Internet is a relatively straightforward operation, and one that does not entail huge costs. Once connectivity has been achieved, the resources on the Internet are just a mouse-click away.

Box 2.3 Minimising your telephone costs

- Always dial your local point of presence.
- Always connect at the fastest possible speed.
- If you can, defer access until off-peak telephone rates apply.
- Plan what you want to do on the Internet *before* you log on, and try to stick to this. Although browsing on the Internet is highly enjoyable (and addictive), be conscious of how much it costs and calculate whether the information you glean is worth the expense.
- Keep FTP'ing of computer programs to a minimum. Programs, by their very nature, tend to be large and therefore relatively expensive to FTP.
- When you have to FTP a computer program (or any large file), try to do this at a time when the Internet is less busy. For UK users this means in the mornings, before the US Internet users have woken up and logged on.
- Configure your Web browser so that graphics are *not* displayed. This will result in Web pages being displayed more quickly, thereby enabling a faster and cheaper Internet session (Appendix B).
- Compose and read e-mail offline.
- Compose and read Usenet News offline.
- Use this book as your offline reference guide.

REFERENCES

1 Net Wizards <URL: http://www.nw.com/zone/WWW/report.html> [Accessed 26 April 1998]

2 Internet Society <URL: ftp://ftp.isoc.org/isoc/charts/networks/overall.gif> [Accessed 26 April 1998]

3 Net Wizards <URL: http://www.nw.com/zone/WWW/report.html> [Accessed 26 April 1998]

4 Digital Research <URL: http://www.research.digital.com/SRC/whatsnew/sem.html> [Accessed 26 April 1998]

5 For details on how to retrieve Web pages via e-mail see 'Accessing the Internet by e-mail: Doctor Bob's guide to offline Internet access' Version 7.2 March 1998. Available at: <URL: http://www.ohio-state.edu/hypertext/faq/usenet/internet-services/access-via-email/faq.html> [Accessed 27 April 1998]

6 Bodleian Library catalogue <URL: telnet://library.ox.ac.uk> [Accessed 27 April 1998]

7 PC Magazine. 1997, 9 Sept. <URL: http://www8.zdnet.com/pcmag/features/isp/ispr5.htm> [Accessed 27 April 1998]

8 Yahoo! <URL: http://www.yahoo.co.uk> [Accessed 27 April 1998]

9 Personal subscription for The Lancet in 1998 costs £95.00 <URL: http://www.thelancet.com/newlancet/sub/arcade/subscribe1.html> [Accessed 27 April 1998]

3

Finding what you want

Box 3.1 Chapter objectives

- Introduce you to the primary search tools now available on the Internet.

- Describe, compare and assess these tools.

- Demonstrate, with practical examples, how these tools can be used to find resources to answer specific medical queries.

INTRODUCTION

Having succeeded in getting your computer hooked up to the Internet, almost certainly the first question you will ask yourself will be: 'How do I find information relevant to *my* needs?' Answering this question is the purpose of this chapter.

At the start, however, it should be pointed out that there is no right or wrong way to search the Internet. Undoubtedly some methods may be more time-consuming than others, but in the end you must choose the method that best suits you. As you come to explore the Internet you will soon appreciate why your Web browser is so named. In my trawls of the Internet I have often come across extremely useful resources simply by browsing and following a series of hypertext links. Essentially though, you can search for information in the following ways:

- by using a **free-text** search engine to interrogate a database of Internet resources;
- by browsing/searching through **subject-arranged** resource lists;

- by browsing/searching through evaluated sources of information.

This chapter will look in detail at each of these and highlight the key strengths and weaknesses of each method. Throughout, the discussion will be punctuated with examples of search questions and descriptions of what was found. Each section will conclude with a 'case study' demonstrating how a specific medical query was answered. These can subsequently be used as templates for any information search you may wish to undertake.

FREE-TEXT SEARCHING

Despite all the hype about the Internet, most users are pleasantly surprised how easy it is to search for information. Both the Netscape Navigator and the Microsoft Internet Explorer – the two most popular Web browsers – have a 'net search' button. Clicking this takes you to a Web page where you can either run a search on a chosen Internet database – Netscape currently points to AltaVista – or you can select another search engine from a reasonably exhaustive list. Either way, searching for a subject simply requires the user to input a word or phrase in the search box and press the 'enter' key. The user looking for information on, say, 'gene therapy' simply enters this term in a search query box and, within a matter of seconds, a list of Internet sites that discuss this topic is displayed.

This function has been made possible by the development of computer programs known as robots. In simple terms, a robot wanders around the Internet gathering details of what is available.[1] Retrieved data is added to a database, which can subsequently be searched. Figure 3.1 shows how users interrogate such a database via a typical graphical query form.

At present there are around a dozen robot-generated Internet databases available for searching. Unfortunately, as these are constructed in different ways, a search undertaken on one and then repeated on another may produce widely contrasting results. The reasons for this are many, but the major factors are that:

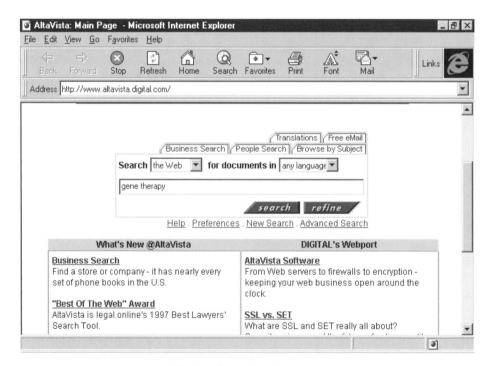

Fig. 3.1 Query–form interface

- some search engines will try and gather everything they find at a Web site, whilst others will collect just a sample of Web pages from any retrieved site;
- some search engines can successfully navigate (and thus index) image maps, frame links and password-protected pages, whilst others cannot.

It should also be pointed out that no matter how big these Internet databases are they do *not* provide an index to everything on the Internet. For example, although a search for 'MEDLINE' will point you to various sites on the Web where you can access this database (Ch. 4), *no* Internet search engine is able to index the data *within* the MEDLINE database.

Detailed below is a practical, quick-reference guide to two of the best free-text search tools currently available.

AltaVista

http://www.altavista.digital.com

The AltaVista database is without doubt the Internet search tool of choice. Its database of more than 100 million Web pages can be searched in seconds, whilst its sophisticated 'refine' features quickly allow you to focus a search to a more manageable number of relevant hits.

Searching the AltaVista database

To search the AltaVista database you enter your term(s) in the query box and press the *Search* button. When the search has been executed the results are displayed in a ranked order, with the most relevant document at the top of this list. The ranking of sites is based on an algorithm that combines the location of your search term on a Web page and the frequency with which that term appears; words in the title section of a Web page are given greater weight than words that merely appear in the body of a page.

A search for 'chronic fatigue syndrome', for example, will find all Web pages in the database that contain this phrase. At the top of the list, however, will be the Web page that has this phrase as its title. When more than one Web page meets this criterion, the frequency with which the phrase appears will be used as a ranking factor. (Note: some Web authors use word spamming in an attempt to promote the position of their page in a Web search. If the AltaVista search engine finds a page where spamming is used it is excluded from the database.)

Even with ranking, the number of potentially relevant Web sites to visit can be daunting. To address this, AltaVista have introduced a feature whereby you can refine a search once the initial results have been displayed. On choosing the 'Refine' option AltaVista suggests related terms which can be added or excluded to the search. Figure 3.2 shows the terms that were suggested as a way of refining a search on 'diabetes insipidus'. In this example, by selecting the terms 'vasopressin' and 'thirst' the number of relevant Web pages was reduced from 1807 to 76.

AltaVista also allows you to restrict the results of a search to a particular language, and through its 'Advanced' search page to limit a search to those Web pages which have been modified during a specific time frame. Special search syntax functions also enable you to search for images, applets, and even how many Web sites have a link to a specific page. Taking this latter example, if I wanted to know how many Web sites had a link to the pages that accompany this book I would perform the following search:

link:www.hbuk.co.uk/kiley/

A summary of the search syntax used by AltaVista is shown in Table 3.1.

Northern Light

http://www.northernlight.com/

A different approach to Web searching is provided by the Northern Light search service. Combining an index to around 50 million Web sites with its own special collection of full-text journal and newspaper articles, Northern Light provides health professionals

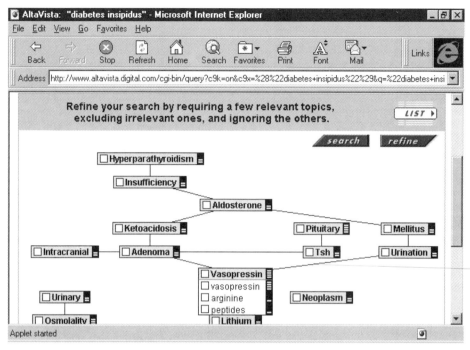

Fig. 3.2 Refining a search at AltaVista

Table 3.1 Search syntax used at AltaVista

Search	Syntax	Example
Phrase searching	Enclose terms in double quotes	"gulf war syndrome"
Combining terms – *both* have to be present	Use the + symbol	+ethics +xenotransplantation
Excluding terms	Use the – symbol	+cancer –prostate
Word stemming	Use the * symbol	gene* (finds genes, genetics etc)
Locating pages that link to other sites	Use the format: **link:**URL	**link:**www.mysite.co.uk
Locating images	Use the format: **image:**name	**image:**gene (finds any image with the name gene)

with a rich and, at times, unique source of information.

Searching the Northern Light database

By default, both the Internet and the special collections database are searched at the Northern Light Web site. The special collections part of the database consists of over 2900 premium sources of information that are not readily available elsewhere on the Internet. Sources indexed within this section include the *BMJ*, *Bulletin of the WHO*, *Chest*, *Journal of Medical Ethics*, *Lancet* and *Pediatrics*. If a search on Northern Light identifies a relevant item from within the special collection then, for a fee (ranging from $1.00 to $4.00), these items can be purchased. If, after buying an article, you decide that it does not really meet your needs you can click on the 'Request a Refund' button, when the fee will be recredited to your account with 'no questions asked'.

In addition to this value-added service, the Northern Light search engine also sorts the

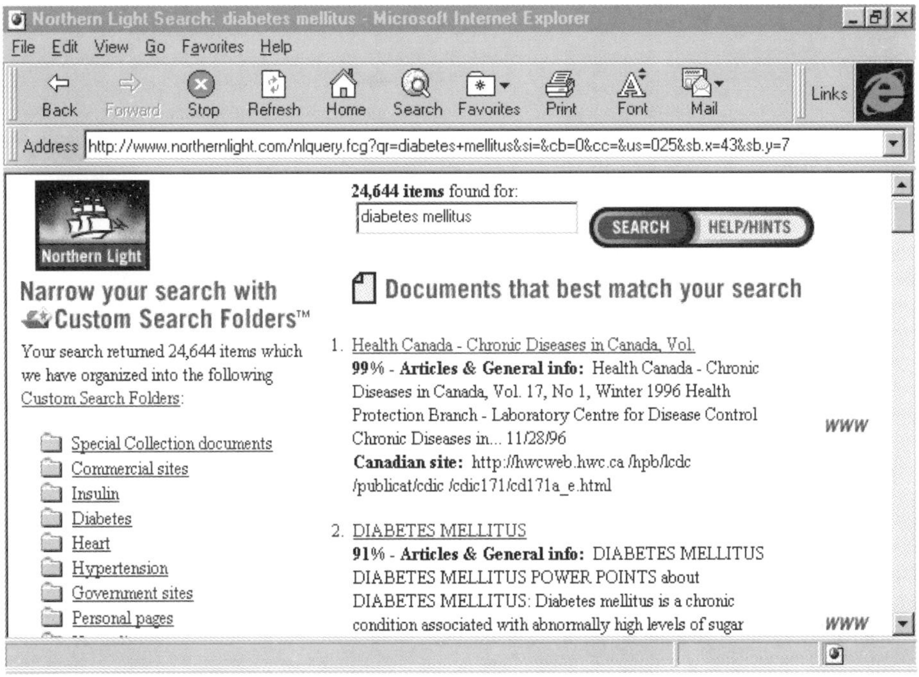

Fig. 3.3 Search folders at Northern Light

search results into discrete 'custom folders' (Fig. 3.3). These folders group like data together based on the subject, source of information (government, commercial, personal pages, etc.), language, and the type of information. At the click of a button you can elect to view, say, governmental sites and ignore all personal Web pages where the data may not be so credible. Within each folder more specific categories are defined, thus enabling you to continually refocus your search.

On searching for information on 'diabetes mellitus' a number of subject folders were identified, such as 'Insulin' and 'Hypertension', whilst domain-specific folders included 'Commercial' and 'Government'. On following the latter category, and limiting this folder to information about insulin, I was pointed to a number of relevant Web pages from sources including the National Institute of Diabetes, Digest and Kidney Diseases[2] and the Healthfinder service.[3] In just three mouse-clicks I had moved from a search that had 24 644 potential leads to one where just 10 Web pages were deemed relevant.

AltaVista and Northern Light: some comparisons

- Because of its size, speed of response and incredibly powerful search options – Boolean logic, supported by date and language filters – AltaVista remains the search engine of choice.

- Although Northern Light tends to identify fewer documents, its ability to sort – on the fly – search results into subject folders is a massive step forward in addressing the persistent problem of 'infoglut'. Moreover, its unique collection of 2 million full-text journal articles ensures that you will find things at Northern Light that you will not find elsewhere on the Internet.

To compare in a more scientific way the relative virtues of both databases, three different types of searches were performed. To ensure that the test was as objective as possible, all the searches were carried out on the same day, and in both databases the default search option

Table 3.2 Comparing AltaVista with Northern Light: a controlled test

Database	Word search "phacoemulsification"	Phrase search "adenosine deaminase deficiency"	Boolean search aldendronate AND osteoporosis
AltaVista	1029 hits	208 hits	2 hits
Northern Light	910 hits	195 hits	5 hits

was used. The results of this test are shown in Table 3.2.

Results analysis

In both the 'phacoemulsification' and 'adenosine deaminase deficiency' searches it was interesting to note that although both databases identified a similar number of hits, the ranking of sites was completely different. Whereas the AltaVista search engine ranked a Web page from the European Society for the Study of Purine and Pyrimidine Metabolism in Man entitled 'Adenosine deaminase deficiency'[4] as the most relevant, Northern Light pointed its users to a page headed 'Modelling workshop for the protein adenosine deaminase'.[5] Both were potentially useful. Moreover, although *many* of the identified sites were common to both, both search engines identified Web pages the other had not.

The Boolean search for information about the drug aldendronate and its use in treating osteoporosis also demonstrated the differences between the two search engines. Of significance, though, was the fact that the Northern Light search identified two items from its special collection, including an article in the journal *Nursing* about FDA approval of this drug and a news item from United News International; neither of these sources is covered by the AltaVista database.

These examples demonstrate the variable results different Internet databases can yield. Consequently, *if* you require an exhaustive and comprehensive search of the Internet you must be prepared to use a range of robot-generated databases.

Strengths of free-text searching

- You can undertake a very specific search and find documents that precisely match your requirements.

- The comprehensive indexing of the retrieved resources means that very few searches fail: no matter how obscure your search there is bound to be a reference to it somewhere on the Internet.
- The databases are easy to search.

Weaknesses of free-text searching

- The non-discriminatory method of document retrieval inevitably produces a number of irrelevant leads. Although a search on the term 'stroke' will point you to useful resources such as the National Stroke Association,[6] the same search will also suggest resources that will help improve your putting *stroke*,[7] and teach you about the workings of the two-*stroke* motorcycle engine.[8]
- The resources added to these databases are not evaluated in any way. For example, if you want to ensure that your *personal home page* can be found by one of these search engines, you can e-mail its details to the AltaVista and Northern Light site administrators.

Using a free-text search engine: a worked example

Box 3.2 is a worked example of how AltaVista was used to find further information about some recently reported research.

Meta-search tools: a brief note

There are a number of meta-search Web indexes that enable you to *simultaneously* search a number of free-text Internet databases. For example, the Dogpile meta-search engine enables you to search 13 Internet databases through one interface. Databases covered by

Box 3.2 Using a free-text search engine: a worked example

Question

A recent newspaper article made reference to a study which showed that a new antiretroviral drug, T-20, can be effective in treating AIDS. Can the Internet be used to help identify this research?

Answer and Methodology

The currency of the information means that the traditional literature searching sources, <u>MEDLINE</u> and <u>Embase</u>, will not yet have indexed this reference; it should, however, be possible to find this research on the Internet. The methodology for this is detailed below:

- Load up a search engine of your choice. In this example, I selected AltaVista. **(http://www.altavista.digital.com)**

- In the search box type in a search concept. In this example, enter the following: +"T-20" +AIDS. (The + symbol means that both terms must be present in the results; enclosing T-20 in double quotes will force AltaVista to search for this as a phrase.)

- AltaVista returns with a ranked list of 181 possible sites. At the top of the list there is a link to *AIDS Treatment News* issue 279, dated September 1997 (Fig. 3.4).

- Select this link **(http://library.jri.org/library/news/atn/atn279.html)**

- At the *AIDS Treatment News* site select the option "T-20: Entirely New Antiretroviral" (Fig. 3.5).

- You are now taken to a brief article which explains the workings of the T-20 drug and the results of a clinical trial. The source of the story – a paper presented at the Infectious Disease Society of America, 35th Annual Meeting in San Francisco (IDSA '97) – is also provided.

Comment

Although the number of jumps may look daunting, it in fact only took just over a minute to reach the news item published in the *AIDS Treatment News*, and identify the full source of this story.

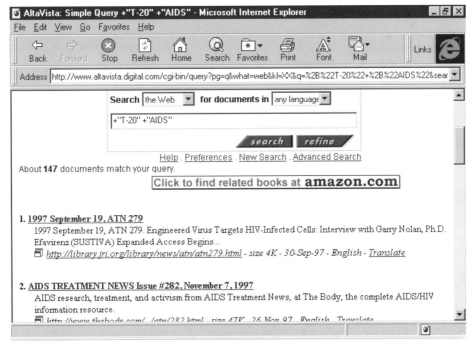

Fig. 3.4 Results of an AltaVista search for "T-20" and AIDS

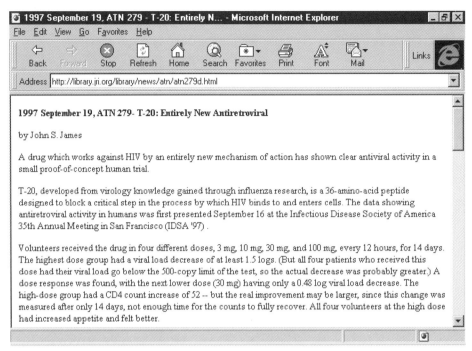

Fig. 3.5 Information about T-20 – from the *Aids Treatment News* Web site

this search tool include AltaVista, HotBot and Excite.

Supporters of meta-search engines argue that by utilising multiple search engines the potential for finding information is much greater. Although this is indeed true, the downside of this equation is that far too many resources are identified and, as you start to sift the results, you naturally find numerous duplicates. Furthermore, as these search tools have to contact a number of databases, the time taken for any search to be executed can be considerable.

The only occasion I can recommend using them is if you are searching for something that is very obscure or rare, and you do not want to manually visit a number of search tools and rekey your search. Table 3.3 lists a number of meta-search tools and their key features.

SUBJECT DIRECTORIES

In many ways the free-text search engines described above can be likened to the index of a book. When you wish to identify precisely where in the text a specific term or concept appears, you consult the index. In contrast, when you merely require an overview of what a book is about you examine its contents page. In this analogy, the subject directories are the contents pages to the Internet.

Thus, the second approach to finding medical information is to browse – or search – through a range of Internet subject directories. These ambitious projects attempt to arrange the resources of the Internet in the fashion of a library. Thus to find material relating to, say, economics, one simply accesses the economics catalogue, where all material on this subject has been grouped.

For medical and health information, the best subject catalogues are the Yahoo health pages and the Biosciences pages of the World Wide Web Virtual Library.

Yahoo! – health section

http://www.yahoo.com/Health
http://www.yahoo.co.uk/Health (UK Mirror)

If the size of the Internet intimidates you, then the Yahoo! site is a very reassuring place

Table 3.3 Meta-search tools: key features

Metasearch tool	Address	Features
Dogpile	http://www.dogpile.com	13 search indexes searchable simultaneously through one interface. Search can be limited to newswire stories.
Internet Sleuth	http://www.isleuth.com	Simultaneous searching of web search engines, directories, review sites and a selection of premier business and financial wire services. Also provides links – and a search form – to 2000+ Web-based databases, including MEDLINE and the NIH Grants Directory.
Personal Compass	http://www.personalcompass.com	Allows you to search 11 search engines or subject directories plus two other meta-search indexes. User can select which search engines to use and save these settings for future use. Results displayed in multiple windows.

to begin a search for information. Here, *all* of the resources within the Yahoo! database are classified within 14 subject headings, one of which is Health.

On selecting 'Health', Yahoo! begins to reveal its tight hierarchical structure. No documents are presented to the user at this broad-concept level. Instead, Yahoo! simply displays another menu, where you select a more specific subject heading from a choice of around 40 topics. These include 'Medicine', 'Nursing' and 'Diseases and Conditions'. On opting for the 'Diseases' section, Yahoo! returns with yet another menu, this time inviting you to select which specific disease you are interested in.

This approach of working from the broader to the narrower concept, continues until no further subdivisions are applicable. When this point is reached a list of relevant sites is displayed. Figure 3.6 displays the links available from the 'Breast Cancer' page. This page is accessed by following the hierarchical links

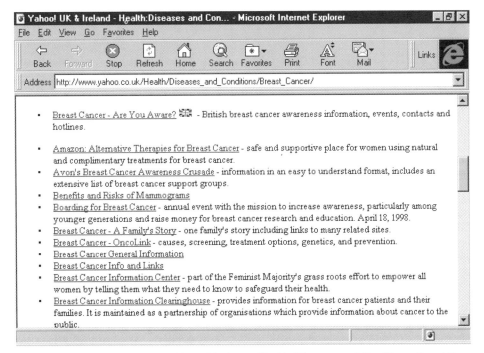

Fig. 3.6 Yahoo!: Breast cancer – the hierarchical route Health: Diseases and Conditions: Breast Cancer

'Health', 'Diseases and Conditions' and 'Breast Cancer'.

If you do not know where a particular subject may fit within the classification scheme you can search the Yahoo! catalogue through its subject search engine. From the results, you can jump to the appropriate part of the subject catalogue.

By virtue of the fact that Yahoo! always displays the subject heading in relation to its position in the hierarchy, you can decide whether to pursue the suggested links or, if you feel that you have been *too* specific in your search, move back up the hierarchy. Continuing with the breast cancer example mentioned above, it is possible that useful links might have been indexed under the 'Cancer' page. Simply by jumping back up the hierarchy, it is possible to go to the authoritative OncoLink,[9] and the National Cancer Institute,[10] both of which have numerous documents relating to breast cancer.

A survey conducted by the market research company RelevantKnowledge identified Yahoo! as the most 'highly trafficked site on the Web', with 26 million users accessing this search index in January 1998.[11] For a quick, user-friendly guide to health resources on the Internet, Yahoo! is certainly worth looking at.

World Wide Web Virtual Library

http://vlib.stanford.edu/Overview.html
http://www.mth.uea.ac.uk/VL/
Overview.html (UK Mirror)

The Virtual Library is the oldest catalogue of Web resources. Unlike other subject indexes and search engines, the Virtual Library takes the form of a *distributed* catalogue, where volunteers take responsibility for identifying resources relevant to their specialty.

Like Yahoo!, resources at the Virtual Library are arranged hierarchically. Thus, within the Biosciences page there are links to more specific indexes, such as Genetics, Neurobiology and Medicine. Within the latter category further specialties are identified, such as AIDS, Nursing and Pharmacy.

As each 'virtual library' is the responsibility of a volunteer, there is little uniformity in the way data is displayed and the currency of these catalogues varies tremendously. For example, the virtual library devoted to Pharmacy arranges the resources into various categories, such as pharmaceutical companies and pharmaceutical databases. Looking at this index in February 1998, one can see that it has been updated within the past 4 weeks. In contrast, the Medicine library is simply an alphabetical list – by provider – of resources related to medicine, which has not been updated since January 1996.

Despite these limitations, the Virtual Library subject catalogues give you a flavour of who is publishing on the Web and what kind of material is currently available. Moreover, if there is a virtual library specific to your discipline you will be pointed to resources other, more general, indexes would not find. Figures 3.7 and 3.8 show sections of the Pharmacy and AIDS virtual libraries.

Strengths of subject catalogues

- Subject catalogues allow you to identify Internet resources from a broad subject base, thereby negating the need to identify highly specific search terms.

- Their hierarchical and browseable structures provide a logical and accessible route to the Internet and thus are an ideal starting point for the new user.

Weaknesses of subject catalogues

- As the creation of a subject heading requires *some* human input, the catalogues tend to be smaller and less up to date than their free-text equivalents.

- Relevant resources may be overlooked by the inappropriate use of subject headings. For example, the premier Internet site for disease prevention, the Centre for Diseases Control and Prevention (CDC), is located in the Yahoo! catalogue only under the obscure and missable 'Government – Executive Branch – Departments and Agencies – Department of Health and Human Services' subject heading.

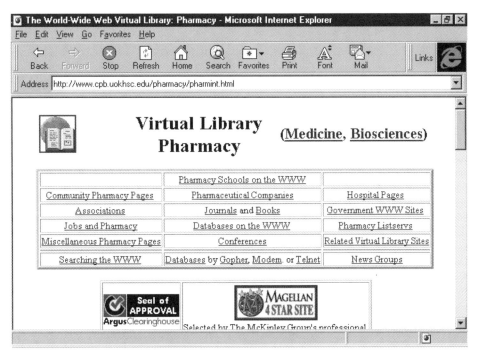

Fig. 3.7 Pharmacy Virtual Library

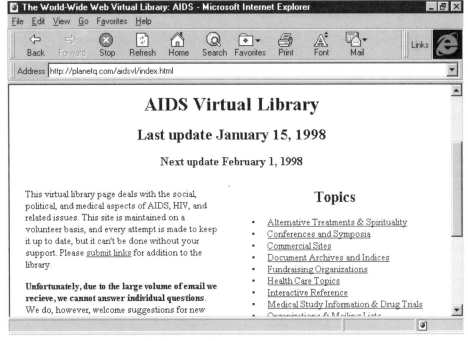

Fig. 3.8 AIDS Virtual Library

Box 3.3 Using a subject catalogue: a worked example

Question

A midwife, on reading that the Internet has resources that are of use to all health professionals, wants to know what is available in the general area of midwifery.

Answer and Methodology

As this is such a general enquiry the free-text databases that search for individual Internet resources will not be of great use. Although one could search for the term 'midwifery' it is likely that potentially relevant sites will be overlooked. A resource on breastfeeding, or caesarean section, for example, that may be of interest to the midwife would be missed if these sites did not include the specific word 'midwifery'. Consequently, a better approach is to use an Internet subject catalogue. The methodology and results are described below.

- Call up the subject catalogue of your choice. I selected Yahoo!, as it is the easiest one to use:
  http://www.yahoo.co.uk/

- From the 'Health' subject category follow the links to 'Nursing' and then 'Midwifery'. If you did not wish to navigate this hierarchy you could search Yahoo! to see if the term 'Midwifery' existed in the subject catalogue. Either way you end up at the same point.

- From the 'Midwifery' subject category, 14 Internet resources are suggested (Fig. 3.9). These range from very specific resources, such as the St Bartholomew School of Nursing and Midwifery, where you can read about their midwifery courses, to more general sites such as the 'Online Birth Centre', where numerous resources of interest to practising midwives can be found.

  If your Web browser has been set up to read Usenet News articles, Yahoo! also includes a link to the *sci.med.midwifery* newsgroup. Following this link will enable you to browse through the recent discussions that have taken place in this midwifery-focused newsgroup. Chapter 6 gives further details of Usenet News.

Comment

Although the resources identified in this search do not represent the total of all midwifery resources, they nevertheless provide the midwife with an excellent starting point.

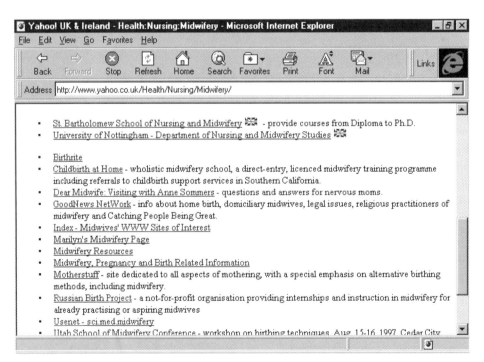

Fig. 3.9 Midwifery resources at Yahoo!

Using a subject catalogue – a worked example

Box 3.3 is a worked example of how a subject catalogue was used to find information relating to midwifery.

EVALUATED SUBJECT CATALOGUES

The third approach you can use to find medical information is to browse, or search, the growing number of *evaluated* Internet subject catalogues. These have been compiled by individuals cognisant with the needs of health professionals who only want to find relevant and authoritative sources of information.

Medical Matrix

http://www.medmatrix.org/index.asp
One of the more established medical search services, the Medical Matrix Project is 'devoted to posting, annotating, and continuously updating full content, unrestricted access, Internet clinical medicine resources'.

Compiled by the Internet Working Group of the American Medical Informatics Association, the Matrix currently has links to around 4000 quality-assessed Internet sites, all of which sit within a browseable, hierarchical subject index. The seven top-level headings include 'Speciality and Disease Categorisation', 'Clinical Practice' and 'Education'. Within each section of the hierarchy resources are further subdivided to allow the user the opportunity to focus the enquiry. For example, resources within the 'Obstetrics' section are divided into categories such as 'News', 'Decision Tools', 'Textbooks' and 'Practice Guidelines'.

In addition to providing the hypertext link to reach the identified resources, the Matrix also gives a description that details what type of information is held at each site. For example, within the 'Obstetrics – decision tools' section, three resources are identified (Fig. 3.10). Using the annotated descriptions you can determine which site best suits your needs, thus ensuring you do not waste your time (or Internet bandwidth) visiting sites that are of little use.

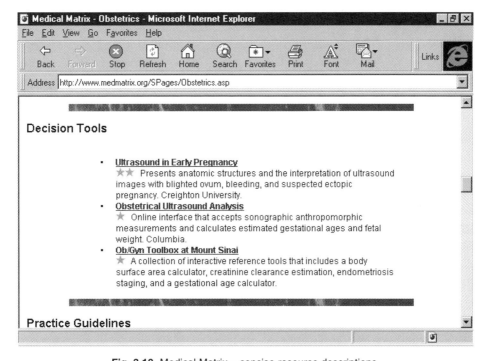

Fig. 3.10 Medical Matrix – concise resource descriptions

Another useful feature of the Matrix is its ranking system. Although *all* the sites within the Matrix meet the basic quality criteria – provide specialised knowledge with suitable clinical content – sites which are deemed to be the 'best of a specialty category' or 'a premier Web sites for the discipline' are awarded merit stars.

Before one can use the Matrix site you must complete a one-off online registration form (the site still remains free of charge). Although form-filling may discourage some users I would urge all health professionals who are keen to find up-to-date, high-quality health resources on the Internet to complete the registration form, and exploit the resources contained with the Matrix.

OMNI (Organising Medical Networked Information)

http://omni.ac.uk

Describing itself as the 'UK's gateway to high quality biomedical resources on the Internet', OMNI is another key resource for health professionals.

Like the Medical Matrix, the OMNI resources database can be both searched and browsed. Recognising the power of browsing, however, the OMNI team have developed an interface which allows the user to browse the database in three ways: by alphabetic topic, by classified topic, and by MeSH (**Me**dical **S**ubject **H**eadings). This latter option – derived from the NLM UMLS metathesaurus – supports broader and narrower relationships, thus allowing far more precise and focused browsing. For example, on selecting the MeSH term 'Eating disorders' you are given the opportunity to elect a more specific term, 'Anorexia nervosa', a broader term, 'Mental disorders', or a related term such as 'Personality disorders' (Fig. 3.11).

To provide a focus for UK Internet resources, the OMNI database supports the option to restrict a search to UK material, a useful feature when so much of the Internet has a US bias. The OMNI site also has details of how resources are evaluated for inclusion in the database, plus a number of excellent articles relating to the quality of health information on the Internet.

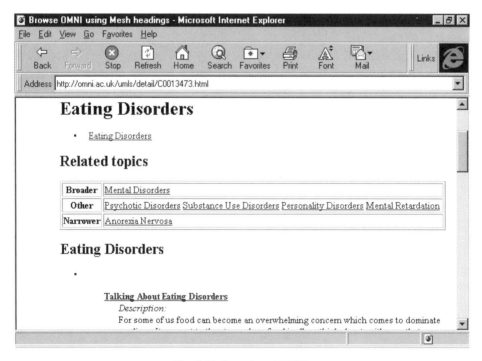

Fig. 3.11 Browsing at OMNI

Health on the Net

http://www.hon.ch/

The Health on the Net Foundation is a non-profit organisation dedicated to 'realising the benefits of the Internet and related technologies in the fields of medicine and healthcare'.

To help realise this objective, the Foundation has developed a *Code of Conduct* for health sites on the Internet. Although this is discussed more fully below (Ch. 7), sites that comply with the Code meet a *defined* quality standard. These 'HONoured' Web sites can be identified by searching the Health on the Net Web resources database (Fig. 3.12).

Somewhat surprisingly, though, this database of Internet resources is *not* limited to sites that comply with the code. Indeed, a search of the database identifies three distinct types of data:

1 Resources which comply with the code;

2 Resources which do *not* comply with the code but have been reviewed by the Health on the Net team;

3 Resources which do *not* comply with the code and have *not* been reviewed. Resources in this section are automatically indexed from 'recommendations' from those Web sites that do comply with the HON code.

Moreover, it would be a mistake to assume that only those sites that complied with the code were worth using. When searching the database for UK resources I found that, although support groups such as Diabetes UK and ADDNet UK are 'code compliant', the *Lancet*, Department of Health and the Medicines Control Agency Web sites are not.

The MedHunt search engine at the Health on the Net site allows you to restrict a search of Internet resources to those that fit within a specific domain – educational, government etc. – or a defined geographical location. It is

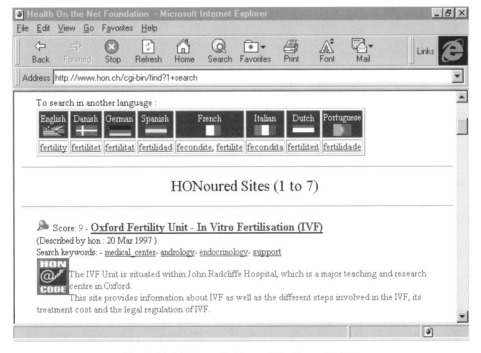

Fig. 3.12 'HONoured' sites – at Health on the Net

also possible to search for hospitals, self-help groups, or for conferences and events.

CliniWeb

http://www.ohsu.edu/cliniweb/

Developed by the Oregon Health Sciences University, CliniWeb is another powerful tool for identifying high-quality clinical information on the Internet.

CliniWeb differs from all the evaluated subject catalogues discussed previously, in that it indexes information at the level of *individual pages* on the World Wide Web. For example, whereas both OMNI and Matrix provide a link to the American Medical Association Web site, the team at CliniWeb have gone further and have indexed individual pages at the AMA site. Thus, a search at CliniWeb for 'tuberculosis' directs you to (amongst other things) an article in the *Archives of Pediatrics and Adolescent Medicine* entitled 'Tuberculosis testing'[12] and an article in *JAMA*.[13]

As with any type of literature searching, the key factor in determining whether or not the search will be successful – that is, retrieve highly relevant documents – is whether or not the correct subject headings are used. To assist in this task, CliniWeb have employed a program called SAPHIRE which maps free-text, natural-language terms to the correct MeSH term. For example, the user can input a phrase such as 'pressure sores', and allow SAPHIRE to map it to the preferred subject heading, 'Decubitus ulcer'.

Appropriate subject headings can also be identified by browsing the MeSH hierarchical structure. Using this method subject headings are made broader or narrower until the desired term is identified. Figure 3.13 demonstrates the hierarchical nature of MeSH on CliniWeb.

The explicit commitment at CliniWeb to include *only* Internet resources that contain clinical information suitable for 'health care education or practice' ensures that searches conducted here refer health professionals to relevant and appropriate information sources.

At the present moment CliniWeb is relatively small. The 10 000 URLs in the database seem

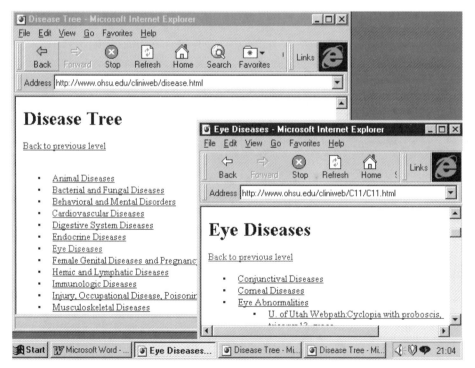

Fig. 3.13 MeSH hierarchy at CliniWeb

insignificant when compared to something like MEDLINE, which, in the last 5 years alone, has indexed more than 1.6 million documents. However, the fact that the CliniWeb developers have decided to index the clinical resources on the Internet at a very detailed level leads me to believe that, in the future, this will also become an invaluable resource for health professionals.

Summary of evaluated subject catalogues

- For a good overview and introduction to evaluated sources of medical information, use the Medical Matrix.
- If you wish to identify quality British resources, use OMNI.
- Use Health on the Net when you wish to restrict a search to a particular domain, or geographic region.
- To identify specific documents, rather than resources of a more general nature, use CliniWeb.

Evaluated subject catalogues: search comparison

Table 3.4 shows the number of Internet resources found when two specific searches were undertaken. All the searches were run on 6 March 1998.

It is interesting to note that although the number of resources identified by these specialised medical search services are of the same magnitude, resources identified by one search service were rarely picked up by a competitor service. Indeed, in the search for resources that discussed 'diabetic retinopathy', all the sites identified were unique; not a single duplicate was found. The conclusion to be drawn from this is that if health professionals want to do a *comprehensive* search for quality health resources on the Internet they must be prepared to use a range of search services.

Strengths of evaluated subject catalogues

- As the resources are evaluated by professionals *before* they are included in the subject catalogue, highly relevant and qualitative sources of information can be identified quickly and easily.
- The short descriptions that accompany most resource entries enable you to decide in advance whether a particular site will provide the information you require.

Weaknesses of evaluated subject catalogues

- Because the catalogues are compiled by individuals, potentially useful resources are overlooked. For example, the Medical Matrix suggests just five resources for the professional interested in migraine. Notable absentees from the list include the JAMA Migraine Information Center[14] and the Migraine Awareness Group Web site,[15] both of which have a large collection of authoritative information.
- Most evaluated subject catalogues are still very much in their infancy, and consequently the number of resources identified thus far is quite small.

Table 3.4 Evaluated subject catalogues: search comparison

Search service	Influenza (no. of resources)	Diabetic retinopathy (no. of resources)	Database size (no. of records)	Date of last database update
Medical Matrix	8	1	4072	6 November 1997
OMNI	14	2	2825	5 March 1998
Health on the Net	6 (452*)	3 (149*)	2500(?)	6 March 1998
CliniWeb	9	6	10000	9 Sept 1997

* These figures represent the sites 'autoindexed' by Health on the Net. They have not been quality assessed

Using an evaluated subject catalogue: a worked example

In Box 3.4 is a worked example of using an evaluated subject catalogue to find clinical practice guidelines on the Internet.

CONCLUSION

This chapter introduced you to a range of search tools available on the Internet. Which tool(s) you use will, in the main, be determined by the nature of the search question and by what you hope to find. When you seek just a few high-quality resources the evaluated subject catalogues will be your best starting point. To get a broader perspective of the information that is available, a general subject catalogue may be of most use. When highly specific resources are sought, a free-text search engine may prove most effective. On other occasions, you may need to use a combination of these tools before you successfully retrieve the information you require.

As the resources on the Internet are so vast you can be fairly sure that no matter how obscure your subject interest is, someone, somewhere, will have posted some information about it. With the tools described in this chapter this information can now be found.

Box 3.4 Using an evaluated subject catalogue: a worked example

Question

A heart surgeon wishes to ensure that the procedures he is following are in line with the best practice guidelines. How can this information be found on the Internet?

Answer and Methodology

Retrieving this information using a free-text search engine would be difficult owing to the large number of potentially relevant search terms: myocardial infarction, cardiac catheterization and thrombolytic therapy are but three potential searches. Although a subject index, such as Yahoo!, would group related resources together, the lack of any defined quality filter means that each suggested resource would need to be individually assessed. A specialised, peer-reviewed Internet medical subject catalogue, however, would overcome these problems.

- Call up the Medical Matrix. I selected this site as all the suggested links in it have been assessed and selected by the American Medical Informatics Association. **http://www.medmatrix.org**
- From the heading 'Speciality and Disease Categorized Information' select the link to 'Cardiology'
- From the 'Cardiology' page select the subheading 'Practice Guidelines'.
- At this page a number of relevant sounding resources are identified, including a database of cardiology procedures compiled by the American College of Cardiology, guidelines from the Canadian Medical Association, the National Institutes of Health and from the UK, 'Cardiology referral guidelines' produced by Eastbourne Hospital NHS Trust (Fig. 3.14).
- Select the link to the American College of Cardiology: **http://www.acc.org/**
- From here you can select from 15 guidelines covering topics such as ambulatory electrocardiography, and the management of patients with acute myocardial infarction. All the documents are dated and are available in full text in either a Web format (html) or as a pdf file (Fig. 3.15).

Comment

This example demonstrates that using an evaluated Internet subject index can be an excellent way of finding relevant and authoritative documents in a very short space of time. From the first link to the Medical Matrix, to the delivery of a number of practice guidelines on your desktop, just five mouse-clicks were made.

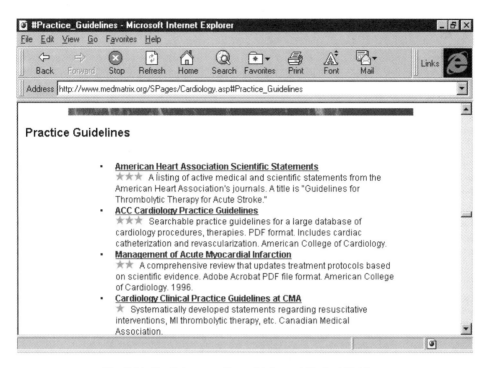

Fig. 3.14 Cardiology practice guidelines at Medical Matrix

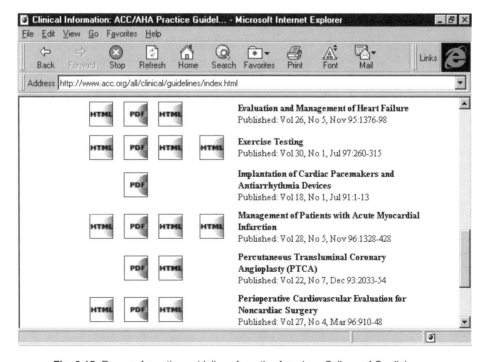

Fig. 3.15 Range of practice guidelines from the American College of Cardiology

REFERENCES

1 A Web robot is a computer program that automatically, and systematically, accesses Web servers to identify what information is available. When this information has been gleaned, the robot moves to the next server.

2 National Institute of Diabetes, Digest and Kidney Diseases <URL: http://www.niddk.nih.gov/ InsulinDependentDiabetes InsulinDependentdiabetes.html> [Accessed 8 March 1998]

3 Healthfinder <URL: http://www.healthfinder.gov/ tours/diabetes.htm> [Accessed 8 March 1998]

4 European Society for the Study of Purine and Pyrimidine Metabolism in Man <URL: http:// www.amg.gda.pl/~essppmm/ppd_pu_ada.html> [Accessed 8 March 1998]

5 Modelling Workshop for the protein Adenosine Deaminase <URL: http://www.isat.jmu.edu/users/ klevicca/isat280/ada.htm> [Accessed 8 March 1998]

6 National Stroke Association <URL: http:// www.stroke.org> [Accessed 8 March 1998]

7 International Golf Accessories <URL: http:// www.2nd-sight.com/products/grips_putting.htm> [Accessed 8 March 1998]

8 Two-stroke engine design and tuning. <URL: http:// www.eric-gorr.com/video_web/ad_2tunvd.html> [Accessed 8 March 1998]

9 Oncolink <URL: http://www.oncolink.upenn.edu/> [Accessed 9 March 1998]

10 National Cancer Institute <URL: http:// www.nci.nih.gov/> [Accessed 9 March 1998]

11 Relevant Knowledge <URL: http:// www.relevantknowledge.com/Press/release/ 02_09_98.html> [Accessed 6 March 1998]

12 Tuberculosis testing <URL: http://www.ama-assn.org/ sci-pubs/journals/archive/ajdc/vol_150/no_7/ oa5369.htm> [Accessed 9 March 1998]

13 Shoe leather therapy is gaining on TB <URL: http:// www.ama-assn.org/special/hiv/newsline/special/ jama/jama313a.htm> [Accessed 9 March 1998]

14 JAMA Migraine Center <URL: http:// www.ama-assn.org/special/migraine/migraine.htm> [Accessed 9 March 1998]

15 Migraine Awareness Group <URL: http:// www.migraines.org/> [Accessed 9 March 1998]

4

The top ten medical resources

Box 4.1 Chapter objectives

- Introduce you to some of the premier health and medical resources on the Internet.

- Provide detailed descriptions of these resources.

- Illustrate by case study how these resources can be used to answer specific medical queries.

INTRODUCTION

One of the best metaphors for the Internet I have come across likened this large and sprawling network to a city. Like any city, the Internet has many useful and interesting places to visit. It also provides opportunities to buy and sell products and, in common with cities, has a seedier and darker side that is best left uncharted.

To find your way around, street maps and signposts are required, which in Internet terms equate to <u>search engines</u> and <u>subject catalogues</u> (Ch. 3). New visitors, however, may wish to supplement their 'A to Z' with a tourist guide that readily identifies some of the best places to visit. With this analogy in mind, this chapter can be seen as your starting point for Internet exploration.

In keeping with the tradition set by all good travel guides every place (site) identified has a map reference – a <u>URL</u> – and a detailed description of the available resources. To keep the discussion focused on how the Internet can help in your day-to-day clinical work, the descriptions of every site also include a case study demonstrating how a specific medical query was answered by that resource.

By providing this information in an offline format, this chapter will help you identify useful resources before logging on, and help develop your appreciation of the wealth of information that now awaits you.

As the Internet is such a dynamic and ever-changing entity there is always the danger that any resource list will be out of date before it has been published. To minimise this danger, emphasis has been placed on the *type* of information a particular server holds, rather than on specific elements of data. For example, it is possible that the World Health Organization (WHO) may remove the information it currently holds on the incidence of malaria. What the WHO is far less likely to do is to remove *all* the resources relating to statistical information. Thus, if you are seeking global and authoritative statistical data the WHO will still be a good starting point.

ACCESS

The top ten medical resources identified in this chapter can be accessed from the Harcourt Brace World Wide Web pages. This single access point not only simplifies your Internet exploration – by making the typing of long and complicated URLs unnecessary – but more importantly, if any of the URLs cited in this chapter change in any way, the new addresses will be recorded and made available to you from this Web page.

To reach Harcourt Brace's medical information on the Internet page, point your Web browser at the following location:

http://www.hbuk.co.uk/kiley/

It is recommended that you Bookmark this page, or even make it your default Home Page (Appendix B).

SELECTION CRITERIA

The number of medical/health sites on the Internet is staggering. As discussed previously (Ch. 3), even specialised medical subject directories such as OMNI and Medical Matrix point to thousands of sites, all of which adhere to a defined quality criterion. As the purpose of this chapter is to introduce just ten Internet resources I have devised my own selection criteria. Therefore I have :

- given pointers to information providers whose contributions to the knowledge base of medicine has long been recognised as authoritative. The Centers for Disease Control and Prevention (CDC) and the World Health Organization are just two examples of 'publishers' who have made a considerable impact on the Internet;
- included a mix of resources that can be used to answer a variety of information queries;
- included a range of different types of information. Some sites are purely textual, others may have a mix of text, graphics and interactive elements, or be in the form of a database which you can search;
- excluded sites that are not regularly updated;
- excluded Web directories that are in effect pointers to other resources. Thus in this list there is no place for sites such as OMNI or Health on the Net (Ch. 3);
- excluded those sites where an extensive range of browser plug-ins are required for the user to access the information. In my definition a pdf plug-in is acceptable – this has in fact become the *de facto* publishing standard – but the shockwave plug-in is not.

THE 'MEDICAL TOP TEN'

In restricting this list to just ten Internet sites, I have inevitably omitted many valuable resources. Those that *have* made it into this list, however, are, in my opinion, the most useful Internet sites currently available for health professionals, and ones which will be accessed time and time again. They are listed in Box 4.2 in alphabetical order, as further ranking would be invidious.

To demonstrate how the Internet can help health professionals in their day-to-day work, each site has a case study where a practical question is posed and answered.

Box 4.2 The top ten Internet sites

- Centers for Disease Control and Prevention
- Internet Mental Health
- The National Institutes of Health
- OncoLink
- PubMed MEDLINE

- Reuters Health
- RxList – The Internet Drug Index
- TRIP – Turning Research into Practice
- WebMedLit
- World Health Organization

Centers for Disease Control and Prevention (CDC)

Address http://www.cdc.gov/

Description The CDC is *the* site to visit if you are looking for information on chronic diseases, injuries and disabilities, or guidelines on their prevention.

In addition to these sources, the CDC has valuable data on travellers' health, plus full-text access to the *Morbidity and Mortality Weekly Report* (*MMWR*).

Cost Free

Analysis The stated aim of the CDC is to 'promote health and quality of life by preventing and controlling disease, injury and disability'. In addressing this broad agenda the CDC has developed numerous information resources of use and interest to all health professionals. Fortunately, many of the resources held at CDC can be accessed through one sophisticated search tool, known as CDC WONDER.

http://wonder.cdc.gov/

CDC WONDER provides query access to about 40 text and numerical databases. For example, when you select the mortality data set, to retrieve data on the causes of death, you can define your search parameters to include a particular state, race, gender or age. Text databases such as the Prevention Guidelines and the *MMWR* can be searched by keyword.

For information about travellers' health, CDC provide a hypertext map of the world. By pointing and clicking your mouse on a particular country you can identify its current vaccine requirements, details of any prevalent diseases, plus general health and travel advice. This type of information is updated on a regular basis to take account of recently reported disease outbreaks. On viewing this site in March 1998, there was a recent report alerting travellers to an outbreak of Rift Valley fever in Kenya and Somalia and advice on what precautions should be taken to prevent infection.

For an illustration of how this resource was used to answer a medical query see Box 4.3.

Box 4.3 Case study for CDC

Following reports that bubonic plague can be 'imported' by international travellers, a hospital microbiologist has been asked to draw up some guidelines for managing such a scenario.

Methodology
As the CDC is probably the world's leading authority on disease prevention, contacting its Internet site to see if any guidelines currently exist on this topic is a logical step.

From the CDC Home Page there is a link to 'Prevention Guidelines' (Fig. 4.1). On selecting this you are taken to the Prevention Guidelines

Database, a 'comprehensive compendium of all official guidelines and recommendations', published by the CDC. This database can be browsed by title or topic, or it can be searched. On opting for the latter, a search for guidelines relating to 'plague' identifies 22 documents, including a report published in December 1996 entitled 'Prevention of plague: recommendations of the Advisory Committee on Immunization Practices (ACIP)'.[1]

This document can be downloaded and printed, and be used to form the basis of local guidelines on the prevention of plague.

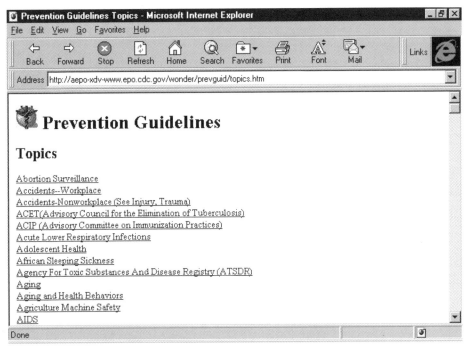

Fig. 4.1 Prevention guidelines by topic – at the CDC site

Internet Mental Health

Address http://www.mentalhealth.com/

Description A one-stop source for authoritative information on mental illness.

Cost Free

Analysis Internet Mental Health describes itself as a 'free encyclopedia of mental health'. Detailed here is information on 52 of the most prevalent mental disorders, supplemented with data on 67 of the most common psychiatric medications.

For every mental disorder discussed, visitors to the site can find a description of the illness, read a synthesis of recent research into its diagnosis, treatment and cause, and be directed to information booklets compiled by professional organisations and support groups. Drug information at this site includes details on adverse effects, contraindications and dosages.

The site also enables you to perform an online diagnosis of a number of disorders including anxiety, eating, mood, personality and those related to substance abuse. Diagnosis is based on the results of a questionnaire you complete while online. Although only a qualified professional can *accurately* diagnose a mental disorder its use as a teaching aid may be considerable.

Note: To undertake an online diagnosis your Web browser must be Java-compatible.

For an illustration of how this resource was used to answer a medical query see Box 4.4.

Box 4.4 Case study for Internet Mental Health

A psychiatric nurse needs to deliver a teaching session on bulimia nervosa to a group of nursing students, and thus requires an overview of the illness, along with information on causes, diagnosis and treatment options.

Methodology
As the literature on bulimia nervosa is vast, the Internet Mental Health site can be used as a source for identifying accurate, research-based information which has been distilled into manageable segments.

Commencing with a definition of the disorder, the Internet Mental Health site provides both an American and European description; the former is derived from the American Psychological Association's *Diagnostic and Statistical Manual* (DSM-IV), whilst the latter is from the World Health Organization's *International Classification of Diseases* (ICD 10). Both manuals provide a set of conditions that must be satisfied before a definite diagnosis can be made (Fig. 4.2).

Following on from this introductory definition, the nurse in this example can then see what research has been published (between 1991 and 1995) in the areas of diagnosis and complications, treatment and cause of bulimia. Each of these sections is in the format of a MEDLINE literature search, with each reference containing the full bibliographic details of the published article and an online abstract.

Additional information about this disorder can be found by following the links to 'Booklets'. In this example there are links to the Royal College of Psychiatrists' Web site and their 'Anorexia and Bulimia'[2] booklet, as well as links to specific pages at the National Institute of Mental Health[3] and the American Psychiatric Association[4] Web sites.

Finally, as a way of adding some interactive component to the teaching session – and to reinforce the information that has been delivered – the students could complete the online diagnostic assessment for bulimia nervosa (Fig. 4.3).

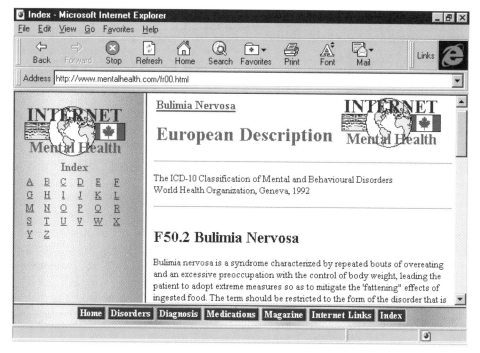

Fig. 4.2 Internet Mental Health – disease definition

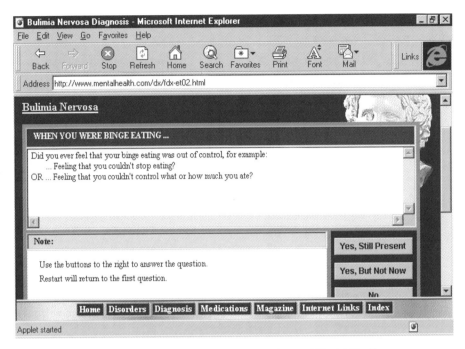

Fig. 4.3 Online diagnostic assessment at Internet Mental Health

National Institutes of Health (NIH)

Address   http://www.nih.gov

Description   Recognised as one of the world's foremost biomedical research centres, the National Institutes of Health provide a range of invaluable sources of information for health professionals.

Cost   Free

Analysis   The mission of the NIH is to 'un-cover new knowledge that will lead to better health for everyone'. It works towards this mission by conducting its own research and supporting the research of scientists throughout the world. Its budget for 1998 was $13.6 billion.

The Web site has links to many health information resources that come under the NIH umbrella. Some of the key links include:

• The Consensus Development Program. The *Consensus Statements* and the *Technology Assessment Statements* that are authored under this program are authoritative guides to current medical issues. Scanning the titles of some of the most recent *Statements* – 'Effective medical treatment of opiate addiction' and 'Acupuncture' – demonstrates the commitment of the NIH to focus on clinical issues.

• CancerNet. Developed by the National Cancer Institute (NCI), CancerNet provides fact sheets on topics such as cancer detection, prevention and therapy. It is also possible to perform a literature search on the CancerNet database to identify references to published journal articles, conference proceedings, government reports and monographs that relate to cancer.

• Office of Alternative Medicine (OAM). With interest in complementary and alternative medicine greater than ever, this is a much-needed resource. The OAM identifies and evaluates alternative health-care practices and disseminates information about them.

• Office of Rare Diseases. A useful resource for identifying information on rare diseases and conditions.

• Grants Information. Details of funding opportunities, how to apply for grants and the CRISP database. This can be used to find details of grants already awarded.

For an illustration of how this resource was used to answer a medical query see Box 4.5.

Box 4.5 Case study for NIH

A general practitioner wishes to run a 'Look after your heart' clinic and seeks some documents that are both authoritative and comprehensible to a lay audience.

Methodology
As the NIH is the umbrella organisation for 24 Institutes and Centres, it is a reasonable assumption that one of these bodies will have a responsibility for cardiovascular diseases and that, once identified, it will have produced some documents that the GP can use. Finding the answers to these questions is relatively simple because the NIH Web site is well structured and easy to use.

Browsing through the NIH Health Information Index, it is evident that the National Heart, Lung and Blood Institute (NHLBI) takes the lead in the

study of cardiovascular diseases. On following the link to the NHLBI Web site a range of resources – grouped by subject – are presented.

Within the 'Cardiovascular diseases' section resources are further divided into topics, such as high blood pressure, cholesterol and obesity. Each of these sections has information for both patients and health professionals. Once you have selected the appropriate subject and readership a number of documents are presented. In this case study relevant pamphlets include 'How to prevent high blood pressure'[5] and 'Controlling high blood pressure: a woman's perspective'.[6] These documents can be printed (or downloaded) and distributed to patients who attend the clinic (Fig. 4.4). Further, provided the source details are retained on the document multiple copies can be printed without any infringement of copyright.

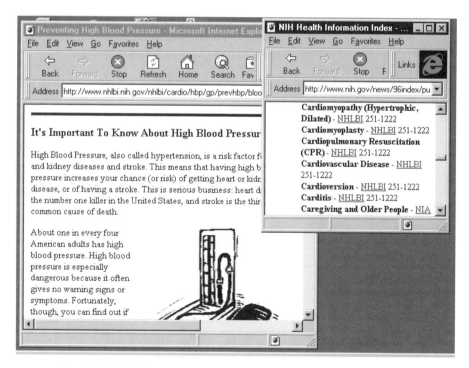

Fig. 4.4 Health Information Index at the NIH – linking to the NHLBI Web site

OncoLink

Address http://cancer.med.upenn.edu/

Description Detailed and authoritative information on all aspects of cancer.

Cost Free

Analysis This site is the only one within this list that is disease specific. Its inclusion, however, reflects the quality of the information and the ease with which cancer-related questions can be answered.

A clear and simple front menu allows you to approach the resources at OncoLink by 10 main categories, including disease, medical specialty (chemotherapy, surgical oncology etc.) and the causes of cancer.

For cancer patients and their families the 'Psychological Support Menu' provides links to documents that discuss how one can cope with cancer, as well as specific issues such as 'Coping with grief and loss'. In contrast, physicians undertaking research on cancer can link to the 'Clinical Trials' section. Here, all trials currently being conducted by the National Cancer Institute and the University of Pennsylvania are cited and discussed.

If the subject you are searching for does not lend itself to this menu approach, the OncoLink search engine can be used. As this uses AltaVista technology (Ch. 3) searching is both familiar and very fast. A search for *+malignant +melanoma +sun*, for example, produces a ranked list of 55 relevant documents.

Perhaps the most remarkable aspect of the OncoLink Web site is that, despite the mass of information held here, it is very easy to find what you are looking for. Cryptic icons are absent, as are labyrinthine hierarchies and browser frames, features that characterise so many Web sites. Developers of new Web sites would be wise to view OncoLink as an excellent example of how information can be effectively disseminated on the Internet.

For an illustration of how this resource was used to answer a medical query see Box 4.6.

Box 4.6 Case study for OncoLink

A health visitor, preparing for a 'Well man's clinic', needs some current information on testicular cancer.

Methodology
Although MEDLINE and other biomedical and nursing databases would be able to assist with this query, a visit to OncoLink may find all the information the health visitor requires.

As this example is focusing on a specific type of cancer, the 'Disease Oriented Menu' option appears most relevant. From this page cancers are divided by age (child and adult) and then by type. Under the adult list, 17 types of cancer are cited, including 'genitourinary (male) cancer' (Fig. 4.5). On following this link a further submenu appears, offering you the choice to retrieve information on penile, prostate or testicular cancer. On selecting the link to testicular cancer a range of resources is presented, including the American Cancer Society's 'Testicular cancer and how to do the TSE'[7] and an OncoLink FAQ on 'Signs and symptoms of testicular cancer'.[8]

To identify additional information, the links to the National Cancer Institute/ Physicians Data Query (NCI/PDQ) database can be followed. Documents in this file are available in a full-text format (not just the bibliographic data) and are tagged to indicate whether the information is aimed at consumers or health professionals. If further information is sought, the results of a number of CancerLit searches on testicular cancer can be accessed.

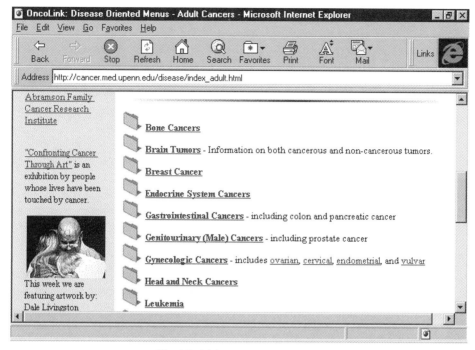

Fig. 4.5 Adult cancers at OncoLink

PubMed – MEDLINE on the Web

Address **http://www.ncbi.nlm.nih.gov/ PubMed**

Description PubMed, developed by the National Library of Medicine, provides a free World Wide Web interface to MEDLINE, the world's premier biomedical database. Dating from 1966, the MEDLINE database currently contains just under 9 million bibliographic citations drawn from around 3800 biomedical journals. In the current MEDLINE file (the last 5 years) 87% of the citations are to English-language sources and 72% have English abstracts.

Cost Free

Analysis Free Internet access to MEDLINE is a relatively new service but one which an increasing number of Web sites now offer. An annotated list of free MEDLINE sites is available at:

> **http://www.medmatrix.org/ SPages/ medline.asp**

Though all these services have unique and useful characteristics, I consider the PubMed MEDLINE to be the best version currently available. The strengths of this service are:

• Currency. By incorporating data from the Pre-MEDLINE file, citations appear in the database far more quickly than in other versions of MEDLINE. Some measure of the currency of PubMed can be gauged by the observations showing that articles published in journals such as *JAMA* and the *New England Journal of Medicine* are indexed – and thus searchable – within one week of publication; articles from the *BMJ* and *Lancet* appear within a fortnight of publication.

• Powerful searching. Using pulldown menus it is possible to search specific MEDLINE fields (author name, MeSH term, title word, etc.) and use the Boolean operators (AND, OR and NOT) to combine search terms. PubMed also has a '*Clinical Query Filter*' that allows you to restrict a search to one of four study categories – therapy, diagnosis, aetiology and prognosis. Once a search has been run and citations selected,

PubMed also gives you the option to find other related articles.

• Links to full-text articles. The NLM is currently establishing links with various publishers to enable MEDLINE searchers to link directly to the full text of a given article. At the time of writing (March 1998) links to around 100 journals, including *Science, New England Journal of Medicine* and *Pediatrics*, had been established. (Note: This feature is publisher specific and users may incur a fee to see the full text of an article.)

• Dynamic links with related databases. A number of MEDLINE articles have links to related databases, such as the Online Mendelian Inheritance in Man (OMIM) database and the Molecular Modelling Database (MMDB).

For an illustration of how this resource was used to answer a medical query see Box 4.7.

Box 4.7 Case study for PubMed

A consultant paediatrician has been asked to prepare a paper on the benefits – or otherwise – of neonatal screening for cystic fibrosis.

Methodology
A search of the MEDLINE database, to identify what has been published on this topic, is the obvious starting point for this enquiry.

At PubMed it is possible to use either a 'simple' or an 'advanced' search form. Whilst the latter enables you to specify specific search fields and incorporate Boolean search statements (AND, OR and NOT) in the search box, the simple form lets you search MEDLINE using natural-language phrases. In this example, as the paediatrician is unsure which MeSH headings and subheadings should be used, the simple search form is selected. The search query is defined as 'screening for cystic fibrosis'. Using the pulldown menu the search is restricted to articles published in the last 5 years (Fig. 4.6).

This search generates 90 results, any or all of which can be selected and printed. On scrolling through the list the paediatrician sees an article by Dankert-Roelse JE, entitled 'Screening for cystic fibrosis – time to change our position'.[9] On selecting this citation further information is supplied – publication type, comments and an abstract – plus links to the *New England Journal of Medicine* Web site and the OMIM database (Fig. 4.7). The link to the journal takes you directly to the relevant article and, in this case, it is available in full text without charge. The link to the OMIM database provides the searcher with a detailed analysis of the genetic makeup of cystic fibrosis. Within OMIM there are links to further sources, including the Human Gene Mutation Database at Cardiff University[10] and the Genome Database at Johns Hopkins University.[11]

PubMed is an extremely powerful search tool and one that exploits the strength of the Web – namely, the ability to link seamlessly from one source to another – to the full. In the example above, the full text of the selected article was just two mouse clicks away from the initial results page. As more publishers recognise the potential of PubMed and begin establishing links with it, PubMed will become an invaluable resource for health professionals.

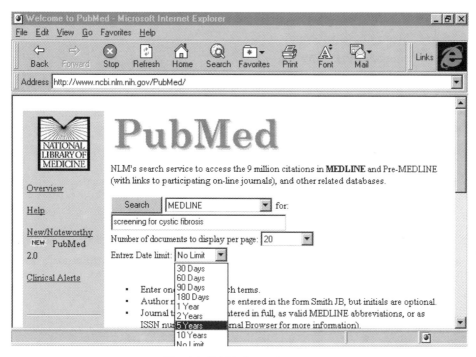

Fig. 4.6 PubMed search screen

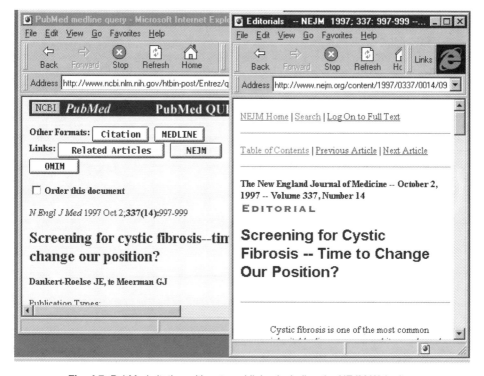

Fig. 4.7 PubMed citation with external links, including the NEJM Web site

Reuters Health

Address http://www.reutershealth.com/

Description A health and medical daily news service keeping health professionals abreast of health stories and scares.

Cost $79.00 per year; $39.00 per year for students.

Analysis Covering around 50 news stories per day, Reuters Health News is the most comprehensive medical news service on the Internet.

To help health professionals find stories most pertinent to their interests, articles are organised into a number of discrete categories, such as clinical, epidemiology and public health. Alternatively, relevant current and archive stories can be identified using a powerful search interface.

All news items cite the original source of the story – typically a research item in a medical journal – and if a story contains a reference to a particular drug, there will be a hypertext link to Reuters Clinical Pharmacology database, where additional information can be found.

Although this is a subscription-based service, visitors can access the consumer health stories (Health eLine) and a number of items from the medical news section every day, without charge. Searching facilities, however, are restricted to subscribers.

For an illustration of how this resource was used to answer a medical query see Box 4.8.

Free Alternative The Medical News pages of the Doctor's Guide to the Internet:

**http://www.pslgroup.com/
   MEDNEWS.HTM**

has a reasonably comprehensive news coverage which, if you wish, can be sent to your electronic mailbox on a weekly basis. Searching of the news archive is also possible at this site.

Box 4.8 Case study for Reuters Health

A patient contacts her general practitioner requesting further details of a story, heard on the radio a couple of days ago, that sudden infant death syndrome may be related to air travel.

Methodology
For topical information such as this, the Reuters Health site will always be a good starting point.
   With so many news stories covered by Reuters it makes sense to search – rather than browse – the news archive. A search for SIDS (sudden infant death syndrome) identifies 64 stories. For convenience these are sorted by date, with the most recent displayed first. In this example, the news item at the top of the list, 'Infants may be affected by high altitude', sounds most promising (Fig. 4.8). On following this link you can read a detailed synopsis of the study and, more importantly, identify the original source of this story[12] (Fig. 4.9).

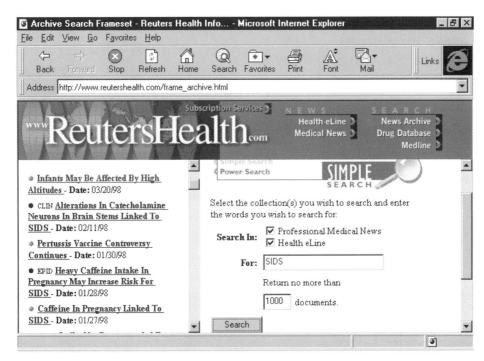

Fig. 4.8 Searching the Reuters Health news archive

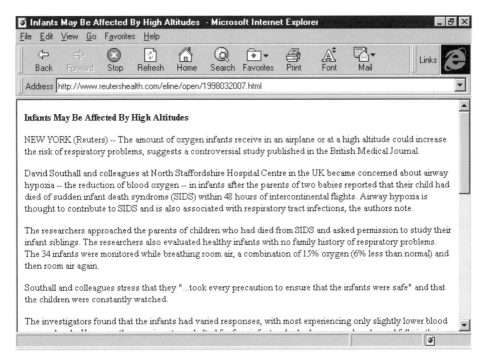

Fig. 4.9 News story at Reuters Health

RxList – the Internet drug index

Address http://www.rxlist.com

Description A database of prescription pharmaceuticals.

Cost Free

Analysis RxList, the 'Internet drug index', provides information on 4000+ prescription drugs. Drug information can be found by either searching the database – by brand or generic name, imprint code or drug category – or by browsing the 'Top 200' prescription drugs. (The top 200 represent 66% of all prescriptions filled in the United States in 1997.) When searching by brand, US names as well as 'foreign' ones can be searched for.

Basic prescribing data is supplemented with 300 RxList monographs. These detailed reports describe key features such as contraindications, adverse effects and drug interactions.

For an illustration of how this resource was used to answer a medical query see Box 4.9.

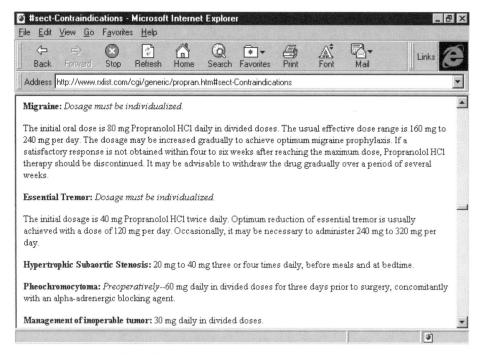

Fig. 4.10 RxList – data on propranolol hydrochloride

Box 4.9 Case study for RxList

A general practitioner, about to prescribe propranolol to a migraine sufferer, wishes to check the literature to ensure that this drug will not interact in any adverse way with the other medication the patient is taking.

Methodology
In a case such as this, the currency and accuracy of the information are the overriding concerns. As the RxList database is updated regularly, and recognised as a source of unbiased information, using this product makes good clinical sense.[13]

The search for 'propranolol' is automatically translated by the database search software to the preferred generic term 'propranolol hydrochloride'. Clicking on this link delivers to the desktop a detailed report, dated December 1997. Information cited here includes a description of the drug, details on usage, and drug interactions. As this drug can be used to treat a wide range of medical conditions information on dosage and administration is arranged according to the condition being treated (Fig. 4.10).

Thus, in a matter of seconds the GP can be reassured, from the evidence that currently exists, that the prescription he is about to write is clinically valid.

TRIP – Turning Research into Practice

Address http://www.gwent.nhs.gov.uk/trip/test-search.html

Description A searchable index to 18 premier evidence-based medicine (EBM) resources.

Cost Free

Analysis One of the problems facing the clinician who wishes to practise evidence-based medicine (EBM) is the disparate way research findings are disseminated. Although the Cochrane Database

(http://www.cochrane.co.uk/abstracts)

is the best source for identifying the results of systematic reviews, other sources, such as clinical practice guidelines and briefing papers, may also be of interest. Finding this information can, however, be extremely time-consuming.

In recognition of this, the Primary Care Clinical Effectiveness Team for Gwent have created the TRIP database, a single searchable index to a range of EBM resources. From this one site over 1550 EBM topics can be accessed. Sources indexed by TRIP include the Cochrane Database of Systematic Reviews, Canadian Clinical Practice Guidelines Infobase, Database of Abstracts of Reviews of Effectiveness (DARE) and the evidence-based health-care journals *Bandolier* and *Evidence Based Medicine*.

For an illustration of how this resource was used to answer a medical query see Box 4.10.

Box 4.10 Case study for TRIP

A neurologist wishes to check that the local clinical guidelines for managing patients with Parkinson's disease conform with the best clinical evidence.

Methodology
Although a MEDLINE search could be undertaken to help try and answer this question, a more focused search, and one that will only identify research that is evidence based, can be achieved by searching the TRIP database.

Using the keyword 'Parkinsons' a search of TRIP identifies nine evidence-based studies.

Included in the results is a study from the ACP Journal Club that compares the therapeutic value of levodopa against levodopa combined with selegiline,[14] a *Bandolier* article that gives a synopsis of recent research on the treatment of Parkinson's[15] and research from the DARE database that examines the effectiveness of the neurosurgical procedure posteroventral pallidotomy (PVP) in managing Parkinson's disease[16] (Fig. 4.11).

All relevant reports can be downloaded or printed and, where appropriate, be incorporated into new, evidence-based practice guidelines.

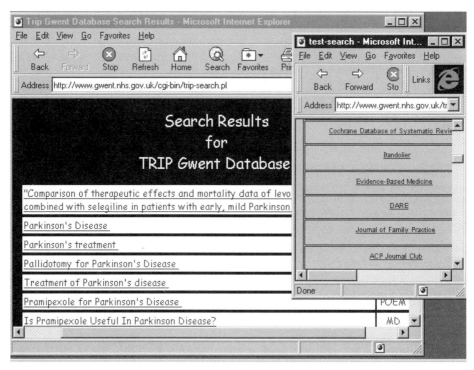

Fig. 4.11 Evidence-based studies on Parkinson's disease – with details of some of the sources indexed by TRIP

WebMedLit

Address **http://www.webmedlit.com/**

Description WebMedLit provides health professionals with a way of keeping up to date with research published in a number of quality medical journals, including *BMJ*, *JAMA* and the *NEJM*.

Cost Free

Analysis Describing itself as a 'medical headlines service', WebMedLit scans the Web every day for updates to the 23 medical titles it is currently tracking. For example, the *BMJ*, published on a Friday, is picked up by this service and is indexed and searchable by Saturday morning. Articles remain in the WebMed-Lit database for around 6 weeks. After this time they should be

retrievable at the PubMed MEDLINE site (see above).

What differentiates WebMedLit from the countless other Web sites providing links to medical journals is its citation database. This gives users the opportunity to search the contents of these 23 journals from one source, *and* the functionality to link directly back to the article (or abstract) at the individual journal's Web site.

As an alternative to searching the WebMedLit database, the latest medical literature can be viewed by subject. Ten general subjects have been defined, including AIDS, cardiology, and cancer.

For an illustration of how this resource was used to answer a medical query see Box 4.11.

Box 4.11 Case study for WebMedLit

A senior house officer has been asked to introduce a piece of recently published research at the next meeting of the Journal Club.

Methodology
With an interest in respiratory medicine the SHO is keen to identify some current research in this area. Less keen, however, is the SHO's desire to visit the local medical library and manually scan through a number of current journals. The WebMedLit site is the preferred solution to this dilemma.

Although the defined subject areas at WebMedLit are too broad for this enquiry, a search of the citation database for 'respiratory tract infections' is undertaken (Fig. 4.12). From this search a number of potentially relevant articles are identified, including one in a recently published issue of *JAMA* entitled 'Antibiotic prescribing for children with colds, upper respiratory tract infections, and bronchitis'[17] (Fig. 4.13). Following the hypertext link the SHO is taken to the appropriate section of the *JAMA* Web site, where the article is available in full text. In this instance an accompanying editorial has also been written.

The WebMedLit service not only negates the need to manually scan a number of key journals to keep up to date in a particular subject, but it also eliminates continual Web surfing to keep abreast of the current medical literature. Further, access to the latest journal issue is not subject to the vagaries of the postal service, or of titles 'going missing' from medical libraries. Finally, if the article you require *is* available in full text there is no need to photocopy it for your colleagues. Instead, all members of the Journal Club simply need to be notified of the appropriate URL.

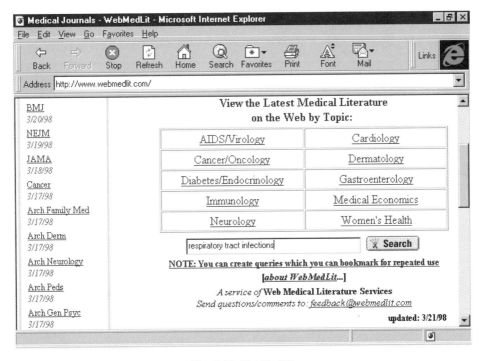

Fig. 4.12 WebMedLit

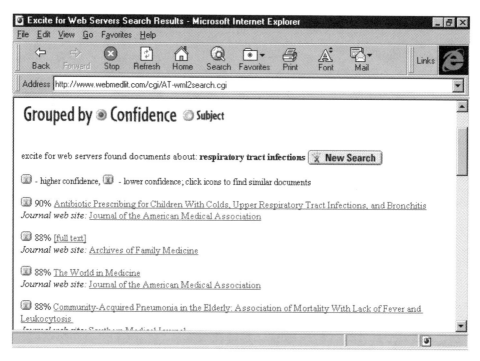

Fig. 4.13 Results of search on WebMedLit

World Health Organization

Address http://www.who.ch/

Description Details of WHO programmes (Global Programme for Aids, Global Programme for Vaccine and Immunisation, etc.); database of WHO publications; statistical databases; *Weekly Epidemiological Report*; press releases and newsletters.

Cost Free

Analysis In recognition of the importance of the Internet, the WHO has made the *Weekly Epidemiological Report* available via the World Wide Web. This electronic journal provides health professionals with a means of obtaining rapid and accurate epidemiological information, along with details of new disease outbreaks.

To identify subject-specific WHO resolutions, guidelines and journal articles, the WHO Management Information (WHOMIS) can be searched.

The WHO also provides a statistical service (WHOSIS) giving Internet users access to a variety of data sources, such as WHO Global Health for All Indicators Database and the Global Programme for Vaccines and Immunization Incidence data.

If you need a global perspective on health, the WHO Web pages must be seen as *the* essential reference point. For an illustration of how this resource was used to answer a medical query see Box 4.12.

Box 4.12 Case study for WHO

An epidemiologist, undertaking some research into measles, wishes to identify the incidence of this disease across Europe.

Methodology
As monitoring outbreaks of notifiable diseases has always been a function of the WHO, it is likely that its Web site will have some relevant data.

Using the Health Topics Index you can quickly identify the main Web page on the WHO site dedicated to a particular subject. Available topic categories include 'Communicable Diseases', 'Tropical Diseases' and 'Vaccine Preventable Diseases'. The latter has links to pages dealing with yellow fever, hepatitis and measles. Data relating to measles is the responsibility of the WHO Global Programme for Vaccines and Immunization (GPV).

At the GPV pages statistical data – in the form of graphs and maps – is available. Material relevant to this enquiry include the 'Estimated cases and deaths from measles, prevented and occurring, 1996'[18] and the 'Reported measles incidence rate per country, 1996'[19] (Fig. 4.14).

If further data is sought, a link back to the WHO Statistical Information Service and its Expanded Programme on Immunization (EPI) Information System will be of use. (**http://www.who.ch/whosis**) Here, incidence data is arranged by disease and region. A table, showing the reported annual incidence of measles between 1992 and 1995 in all European countries, can be accessed and downloaded.[20]

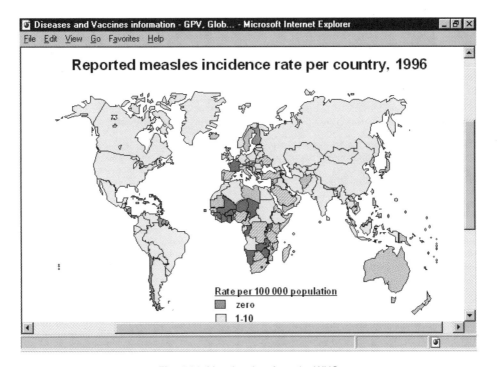

Fig. 4.14 Measles data from the WHO

CONCLUSION

The only way to fully appreciate and exploit the range of resources described in this chapter is to visit these sites and explore. In particular, I would urge you to pay special attention to the *'What's New'* links. Although at times these may simply serve to distract you from your original objective, on other occasions they will bring to your attention new and useful resources which otherwise would have remained undiscovered.

As you trawl the Internet you will undoubtedly discover numerous other sites of interest and effectively compile your own 'top ten resources'. If you would like to share these findings with other health professionals, please e-mail the details to me through the Harcourt Brace World Wide Web pages. Subject to quantity a 'reader's top ten' will be made available there, along with hypertext links to other recommended sites.

REFERENCES

1 Prevention of plague: recommendations of the Advisory Committee on Immunization Practices (ACIP) <URL: http://aepo-xdv-www.epo.cdc.gov/wonder/prevguid/m0044836/entire.htm> [Accessed 25 March 1998]
2 Royal College of Psychiatry <URL: http://www.ex.ac.uk/cimh/help/anorexia.htm> [Accessed 25 March 1998]
3 National Institute of Mental Health <URL: http://www.nimh.nih.gov/publicat/eatdis.htm> [Accessed 25 March 1998]
4 American Psychiatric Association <URL: http://www.psych.org/public_info/eating.html> [Accessed 25 March 1998]
5 National Heart, Lung and Blood Institute <URL: http://www.nhlbi.nih.gov/nhlbi/cardio/hbp/gp/prevhbp/blood.htm> [Accessed 25 March 1998]
6 National Heart, Lung and Blood Institute <URL: http://www.nhlbi.nih.gov/nhlbi/cardio/hbp/gp/hbp_wmn.htm> [Accessed 25 March 1998]
7 American Cancer Society <URL: http://cancer.med.upenn.edu/disease/testicular/tse.html> [Accessed 25 March 1998]
8 Oncolink <URL: http://cancer.med.upenn.edu/disease/testicular/faq/faq_testicular1.html> [Accessed 25 March 1998]
9 Dankert-Roelse JE 1997 Screening for cystic fibrosis – time to change our position? New England Journal of Medicine 337(14):997–999
10 Human Gene Mutation Database <URL: http://uwcm.ac.uk/uwcm/mg/hgmd0.html> [Accessed 1 April 1998]
11 Genome Database <URL: http://gdbwww.gdb.org/gdb> [Accessed 3 April 1998]
12 Parkins KF 1998 Effect of exposure to 15% oxygen on breathing patterns and oxygen saturation in infants: interventional study. BMJ 316 (8135):887–894
13 Medical Matrix – the Internet directory has assigned RxList a two star rating. This is defined as 'a valuable resource for improving general knowledge in the discipline, or other outstanding features, such as multimedia'
14 American College of Physicians Journal Club <URL: http://www.acponline.org/journals/acpjc/mayjun96/levodopa.htm> [Accessed 3 April 1998]
15 Bandolier <URL: http://www.jr2.ox.ac.uk/Bandolier/band23/b23-4.html> [Accessed 3 April 1998]
16 NHS Centre for Reviews and Dissemination <URL: http://nhscrd.york.ac.uk/> [Accessed 3 April 1998]
17 Nyquist AC 1998 Antibiotic prescribing for children with colds, upper respiratory tract infections, and bronchitis. JAMA 279(11):875–877
18 WHO <URL: http://www.who.ch/gpv-surv/map+graph/graphsub/measlescascov.htm> [Accessed 25 March 1998]
19 WHO <URL: http://www.who.ch/gpv-surv/map+graph/mapsub/meainc.htm> [Accessed 25 March 1998]
20 WHO <URL: http://www.who.ch/whosis/epi/inc/m4.txt> [Accessed 25 March 1998]

5

Interactive learning

Box 5.1 Chapter objectives

- Examine how medical education is being delivered over the Internet.

- Provide detailed descriptions of innovative examples of medical education on the Internet.

- Highlight the benefits of using the Internet for medical education.

INTRODUCTION

Alhough the Internet was originally devised for military and defence purposes, it was not long before academics, realising its potential, seized the initiative. Spurred on by a vision of the future, where communication would be quick and simple (e-mail) and where research findings and data could be transferred at the touch of a button (FTP), the academic community began to invest time and money in developing computer networks.

As early as 1979 parts of the UK academic community were linked by a network created by the Science Research Council (SRC) and the National Education Research Council (NERC). By 1984 this network had expanded – and been renamed JANET (Joint Academic Network) – to enable all universities and research laboratories to enjoy the benefits of wide area networking.

Throughout the late 1980s JANET continued to expand as more polytechnics and colleges of higher education sought access. In 1991 the JANET IPS (Internet protocol service) was created. This development meant that everyone on the JANET network could now access all the other computers on the Internet.

As networks have grown and become more robust, academics and other professionals have begun to appreciate how they can be used in the process of teaching and learning. This chapter will examine this development with reference to medical education on the Internet. Specifically, we will look at how the Internet is being used as a medium for delivering:

- virtual interactive patient simulations;
- lecture notes, tutorials and multimedia textbooks;
- online courses;
- examinations;
- virtual conferencing.

For each of these subject areas one *innovative* Internet site will be discussed and assessed. For those who wish to explore further, other sites are recommended.

VIRTUAL INTERACTIVE PATIENT SIMULATIONS

From a patient's perspective the most important skill a doctor should possess is the ability to diagnose illnesses quickly and accurately. Such a talent, however, tends to be acquired more with practice and experience than with theoretical learning. Indeed, it is highly probable that a recently qualified doctor will have had little direct contact with 'live' patients.

In recognition of this problem a number of doctor/patient simulated encounters can now be experienced on the Internet. The best of these are described below.

The Interactive Patient

http://medicus.marshall.edu/mainmenu.htm

Developed by the Marshall University School of Medicine in 1995, the Interactive Patient is an interactive World Wide Web program that allows you to simulate an actual patient consultation. The program begins by presenting the user with an opportunity to take a patient history. Information acquired here can be enhanced with a physical examination and by examining a range of laboratory results and X-rays. When a complete picture of the illness has been constructed you are invited to submit a diagnosis and course of treatment.

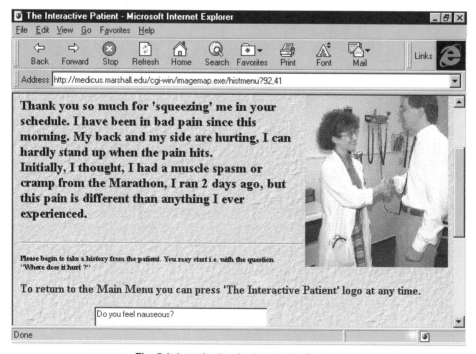

Fig. 5.1 Interviewing the Interactive Patient

What makes this product unique is the way you can directly *interact* with the patient (Fig. 5.1). Thus, from the opening screen, where the patient informs you of a 'pain in his side', the direction the interview takes is entirely under your control. For example, on asking the question 'Do you feel nauseous?', the Interactive Patient replies,

'Ever since the pain started at 9.00 am this morning I have been somewhat nauseous. When the pain gets worse I start to feel sick in my stomach as well.'

Using this answer as a clue to the nature of the illness you can ask a follow-up question, such as 'Have you had any difficulty passing urine?' This questioning continues until you are satisfied that no further relevant information can be gleaned from the patient.

If you ask a question the patient is unable to answer you are asked to be 'more specific'; this reply simply means that the question does not contain any keywords present in the Interactive Patient's database.

As it is believed that around 82% of all outpatient diagnoses are based *exclusively* on what is learnt during the history-taking session, it is essential that considerable time is spent on teaching students how to take full and accurate histories.[1] The Interactive Patient goes some way towards addressing this issue.

Once the history has been taken you then have the opportunity to undertake a physical examination. Options currently available allow you to inspect, palpate or auscultate the patient. If you auscultate the heart (by pointing and clicking your mouse on the appropriate part of the patient's torso), you can actually hear how it sounds (Fig. 5.2). If you do not have a sound card and speakers in your computer to support this function the sound will be described to you. In this example the following message was relayed:

'The heart sounds are regular without murmur. There is a prominent split S2.'

The final pieces of the diagnosis jigsaw are the laboratory results and X-rays. More than 20 laboratory tests have been performed on this patient, ranging from vital signs (temperature, heart rate and blood pressure)

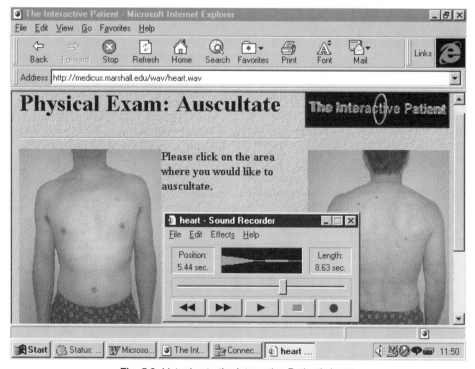

Fig. 5.2 Listening to the Interactive Patient's heart

to a complete blood count, and coagulation studies. For additional clues to the cause of the patient's pain, five radiological investigations have been performed. These include a chest X-ray, a CT scan of the lumbar vertebrae and an abdominal ultrasound.

Laden with this armoury of diagnostic evidence, you are finally invited to submit a diagnosis and indicate which of the suggested therapeutic options would be most effective. Depending upon how busy the Marshall <u>server</u> is, a comment on your diagnosis and treatment is normally mailed to you within the hour.

Once you have successfully completed a case at the Interactive Patient you will receive an electronic message containing an application form for a CME (Continuing Medical Education) Credit Certificate. A CME credit of one hour in 'Category 1 of the Physicians Recognition Award of the American Medical Association' is awarded for completing a case.

Recommended sites for further exploration

Trauma Moulage

http://www.trauma.org/resus/moulage/
moulage.html

Developed by Trauma Org – an independent body that exists to promote and disseminate the knowledge and practice of injury prevention and trauma care throughout the world – the Trauma Moulage pages have been designed to reinforce the basic principles of trauma resuscitation. This is achieved via a number of practice trauma scenarios. In the first moulage the following scenario is presented:

> You are an emergency room doctor and must assess and adequately treat an injured patient. You have an assistant to help you, but they can be of variable help, as in real life.

As you work through the pages further information about the condition of the patient is provided, as are a number of possible options. For example, having decided that the priority is to secure the patient's airway, four

possible options are presented: nasotracheal intubation, orotracheal intubation, cricothyroid puncture or tracheostomy. If you select the appropriate treatment – orotracheal intubation – the scenario continues. If you select an inappropriate treatment, the patient dies.

All of the scenarios are written in a light-hearted and amusing way, a feature which reinforces the learning experience.

Virtual Autopsy

http://www.le.ac.uk/pathology/teach/VA

In contrast to the virtual patient, staff at the University of Leicester have created the Virtual Autopsy Web site, where you have to identify the cause of death in seven autopsy cases. Each case begins with a clinical history, along with supporting data such as X-rays and blood films.

To help identify the cause of death, images of the patient's organs and detailed autopsy reports are presented for analysis. When all the evidence has been gathered you are presented with a list of possible causes. If you get the answer wrong there are additional hints to help you find the correct cause of death. In an educational context this positive approach to error is more effective than the alternative, where you are simply informed that your diagnosis is incorrect.

LECTURE NOTES, TUTORIALS AND TEXTBOOKS

As more and more material relating to medical education is published on the Internet, traditional learning patterns and practices are being swept away. For example, in pre-Internet days if a medical student missed a lecture he would, assuming he was conscientious, be forced to copy up the notes from a colleague. Nowadays it is possible that the lecture notes will be published on the Internet, where they can be perused (or downloaded) at a more convenient time.

Similarly, if a student wishes to supplement the lecture with some additional reading he is no longer constrained by the restrictive opening hours of his local medical library. Via the Internet, various medical textbooks and journals are available. Most strikingly, some of these will be multimedia publications enabling, for example, the student to hear abnormal lung sounds or watch a video of a surgical procedure.

Discussed below are some of the best examples on the Internet of this type of material.

Lecture Notes in Orthopaedics

http://www.worldortho.com/database/
   lectures/lecture1.html

Although there are numerous lecture notes on the Internet, one of the more developed series is the Lecture Notes in Orthopaedics, published by WorldOrtho, 'the ultimate orthopaedic and sports medicine Website'.

Written by Eugene Sherry, Senior Lecturer in the Department of Orthopaedic Surgery, University of Sydney, Australia, the series of six lectures available here is used as part of the official teaching curriculum for medical students at the University of Sydney. Subjects covered include trauma, low back pain and fractures.

The lecture notes are written in a clear concise format and are supported with relevant images. Where available, links are made between the notes and the series of case studies that WorldOrtho also hosts.

Tutorials – The Internet Pathology Laboratory

http://www-medlib.med.utah.edu/WebPath/
   TUTORIAL/TUTORIAL.html

WebPath, a product of the Department of Pathology, University of Utah, is a huge resource for any pathology student or health professional, comprising more than 1900 images, 1600 examination questions and numerous laboratory exercises and tutorials.

Twenty tutorials are available covering topics as wide-ranging as drug abuse pathology, firearms and tuberculosis. The firearms tutorial, for example, is designed to provide stu-

dents with 'a working knowledge of the types of firearms, the types of ammunition used, the nature of injuries that can be produced in the body, and the investigative techniques employed by the forensic pathologist in assessing firearms injuries'. This is achieved by dividing the tutorial into discrete sections, each of which is annotated with appropriate descriptions and images. Figure 5.3 shows the microscopic image of a gunshot entrance wound with gunshot residue. Each tutorial concludes with a series of references for further reading.

Textbooks – Global Textbook of Anaesthesia

http://gasnet.med.yale.edu/gta/
http://gasnet.dundee.ac.uk:1081/gta/ (UK
   mirror site)

The Global Textbook of Anaesthesia is a good illustration of how the Internet can be used to deliver high-quality medical textbooks. Specifically, it is:

- a truly worldwide product. Contributors from Canada, the United States, Germany and Australia have authored various chapters and, on some occasions, taken the responsibility for hosting that section on a 'local' Web server;
- multimedia in content. For example, the chapter on 'Fiberoptic endotracheal intubation' contains a number of video clips that show how this procedure can be performed (Fig. 5.4);
- hypermedia in format, ensuring that you can jump seamlessly from one section to another;
- free at the point of use.

Developed by GASNet, the Global Anaesthesiology Server Network, the Global Textbook of Anaesthesia comprises 14 chapters that cover all aspects of anaesthesia. These include pain management, anaesthetic complications and obstetric anaesthesia. There is also an electronic phrase book – in English, German, Hebrew, Italian and Spanish – that contains a comprehensive list of phrases and

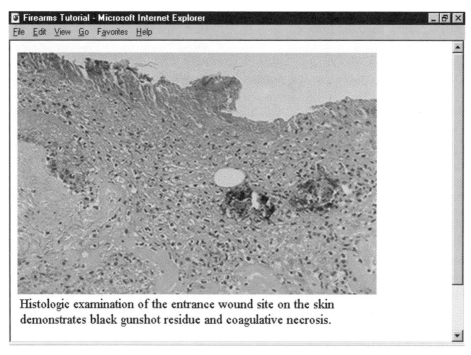

Fig. 5.3 Microscopic image of gunshot wound – part of a WebPath tutorial

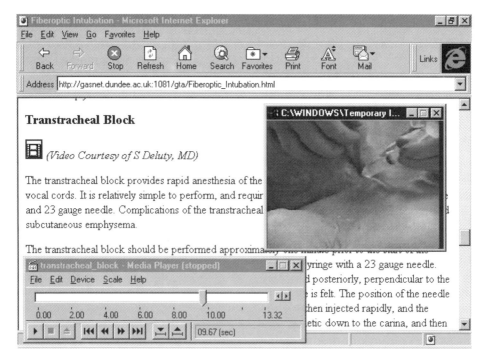

Fig. 5.4 Transtracheal block – a video still from the Global Textbook of Anaesthesia

consent statements that may be useful for anaesthesiologists.

Recommended sites for further exploration

Supercourse: epidemiology, the Internet and global health

http://www.pitt.edu/~super1/main/ lecture.htm

Another good series of lecture notes is that published at the Supercourse Web site. Comprising 33 separate lectures, this site is designed to provide an overview of epidemiology for medical and health-related students around the world. Lectures available include 'Disease monitoring', 'Malaria' and 'Clinical trial concepts'. It takes the format of a slide show and visitors can work through the lectures at their own pace, following any of the suggested hypertext links as appropriate.

Recognising the global nature of the Internet, a number of the lectures are available in a variety of languages: the first introductory lecture is available in eight languages, including Chinese, Japanese and Russian. To ensure that the lectures meet their intended objectives every participant is encouraged to complete an online questionnaire.

Merck Manual of Diagnosis and Therapy

http://www.merck.com/

Believed to be the 'most widely used medical textbook in the world',[2] the 16th edition of the Merck Manual of Diagnosis and Therapy (1992) is available in full text at the Merck Web site. (The 17th edition will be available in early 1999.)

The Manual can be browsed by section – infectious diseases, pulmonary disorders etc. – or it can be searched (Fig. 5.5). A search on 'aortic stenosis', for example, directs you to the section within the cardiovascular disorders, and also to the paediatrics and genetics chapter, where there is a section on congenital abnormalities.

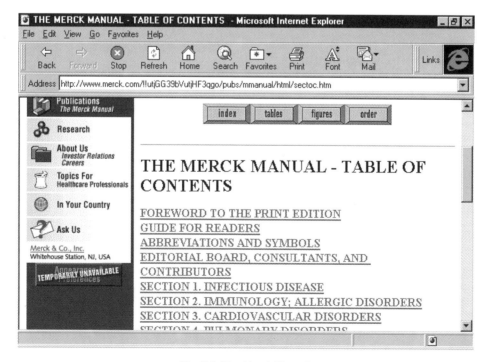

Fig. 5.5 The Merck Manual

Virtual Hospital

http://www.vh.org/Providers/Textbooks/
MultimediaTextbooks.html

The Virtual Hospital defines itself as a 'continually updated digital health sciences library' providing information to both patients and health-care providers 24 hours a day. With regard to this latter group, the Virtual Hospital identifies the need to provide distance learning facilities as one of its primary objectives. The provision of high-quality, up-to-date, multimedia medical textbooks is one way this objective is currently being addressed.

Twenty-five such texts, commissioned by the Virtual Hospital, are now available from this site. Topics covered range from muscle and back injuries, through to pulmonary embolus and treatment of congenital club foot.

ONLINE COURSES

For those students who require more than a read-only, hypertext tutorial, interactive online courses are now being developed for the Internet. One such course that may be of interest to the medical community is the *Online BioComputing Course.*

Online Course in BioComputing

http://www.techfak.uni-bielefeld.de/bcd/
welcome.html

Run by the Virtual School of Natural Sciences, this 10-week course offers students a 'profound introduction to biosequence analysis and comparison'.

Although the entire course is conducted over the Internet – thereby enabling you to follow it from your own home – in all other respects it takes the same format as any course you may attend at a university or college. Thus, students are required to participate in discussion forums, work in groups and undertake individually assigned coursework. Completed assignments are transmitted for marking and comment by e-mail, whilst discussion and group work is facilitated by the virtual meeting place, <u>BioMOO</u> (see below).

This course has now been run twice and has attracted students and speakers from all parts of the world. Plans are now in hand to recruit students for the next course.

Recommended sites for further exploration

Diploma of Health Informatics – University of Otago, New Zealand

http://corriander.otago.ac.nz:800/

This postgraduate course is being run jointly by the Wellington School of Medicine and the Department of Information Science of the University of Otago, New Zealand.

In true distance learning style all assignments are submitted via e-mail, whilst discussions with colleagues and tutors are conducted via an Internet discussion list. Where a live and interactive forum is required – for tutorials and group discussions – <u>Internet Relay Chat</u> is the preferred medium.

Although at the present time access to this course is restricted to students resident in New Zealand, there are plans to remove this restriction in the near future.

CASO's Internet University

http://www.caso.com/

To identify other online courses in other disciplines, the CASO's Internet University Web site can be consulted. This one site lists more than 2500 Internet-based courses – from over 80 accredited course providers – and provides details such as who the course is aimed at, the mode of teaching, and the number of educational credits each course attracts. Figure 5.6 shows some of the courses arranged within the 'Health' category.

ONLINE EXAMINATIONS

Preparing for examinations is almost a way of life for recently qualified medical staff. In the UK, this takes the form of preparing for Part I and Part II of the Membership and Fellowship

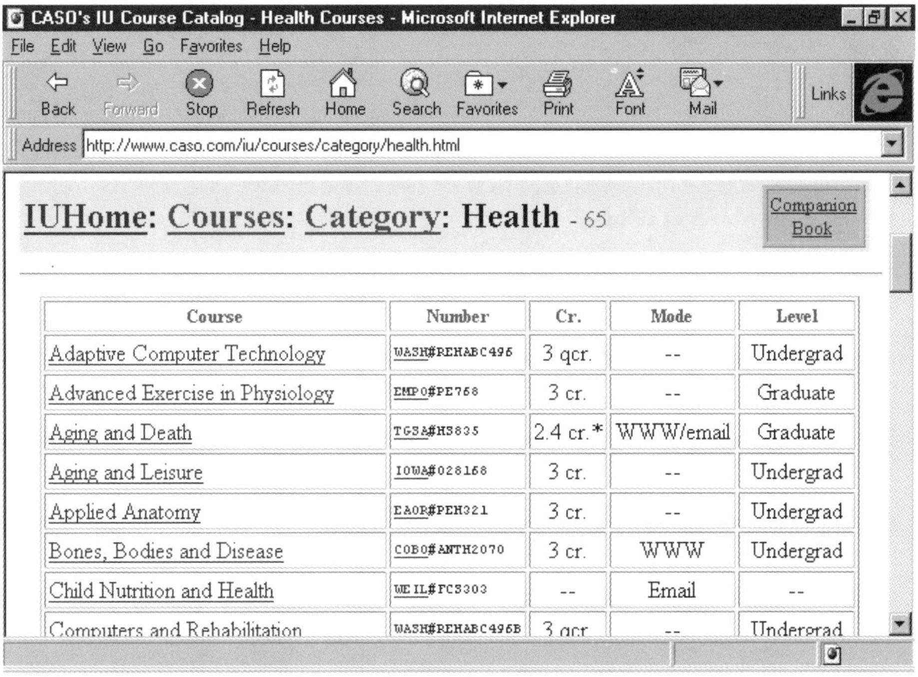

Fig. 5.6 Directory of online courses from the Internet University

examinations, organised by the various Royal Colleges.

Although some information about these examinations – dates, fees, eligibility etc. – is available at each of the awarding bodies' Web sites,[3] absent from these pages are any past examination papers which could help candidates prepare more effectively. One 'unofficial' site that goes some way towards addressing this issue is the MRCP Part I Question Bank, created by Dr Dean Jenkins, Specialist Registrar at Llandough Hospital, Cardiff.

MRCP Part I Question Bank

http://homepages.enterprise.net/djenkins/mcqs

Consisting of 900 questions – of the type seen in the MRCP Part I examination – students can either work through the entire question bank or, if they feel they are weaker in a particular area, run a search against the database to identify questions on a particular sub-

ject. The answer(s) to each question, along with explanatory comments, is revealed by mouse-clicking the 'answer' box (Fig. 5.7).

Recommended sites for further exploration

X-Ray Files

http://www-ipg.umds.ac.uk/~acd/xrayfiles/index.htm

Students preparing for Part I of the Fellowship of the Royal College of Radiologists (FRCR) will find the X-Ray File Web site particularly useful. Created and maintained by Dr Downie, of the United Medical and Dental Schools of Guy's and St Thomas's Hospital, this site contains a mix of multiple-choice questions and radiological case studies.

Professionals who have advanced beyond Part I of the FRCR can turn to the more complex tutorials and case studies.

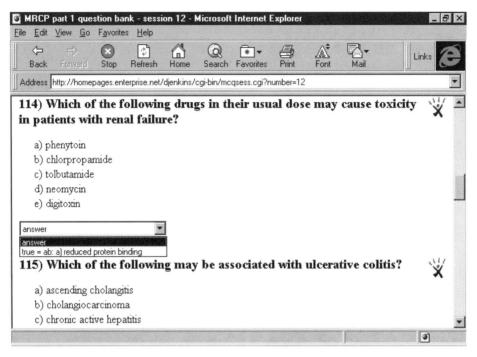

Fig. 5.7 MCQ preparation for the MRCP Part I examination

MedWeb Automated Assessment Service

http://medweb.bham.ac.uk/http/caa/newdb/

Developed by the University of Birmingham Medical School, the Medweb Automated Assessment Service (MAAS) provides medics with a further opportunity to practise answering MCQs.

Visitors to this site can answer questions from a preset quiz, or alternatively devise their own quiz by searching for questions in the database that match a user-defined keyword. Either way, the MAAS will automatically mark your answers and give a score and feedback on your performance, as appropriate.

VIRTUAL CONFERENCING

A study conducted in 1988 on continuing education for General Practitioners[4] found that the main reasons for attending continuing education meetings were:

- they provided new information and reminders of things that were already known;
- they provided a useful means of meeting other general practitioners and consultants, and thus provided a forum where common problems could be discussed.

In contrast, reasons for non-attendance included:

- lack of time;
- inconvenient meeting time;
- venue too far away.

Although in more recent years the GP Contract, with its concomitant educational allowance, has added a financial incentive for attending educational meetings, the reasons identified for non-attendance are still valid.

Through the Internet, however, it is possible to enjoy the benefits of peer discussion and analysis *without* the trouble of attending some distant postgraduate centre. This dream-like scenario is made possible by the 'virtual conference', where physical attendance at a meeting is replaced by a virtual presence through your computer. BioMOO is the best example at the moment of a virtual meeting place.

Also, an increasing number of major international medical conferences transmit some of their proceedings over the Internet. Specific examples are discussed here and pointers are given to help you identify future online conferences.

BioMOO

**http://bioinformatics.weizmann.ac.il/
BioMOO/**

BioMOO is a text and image-based virtual reality system for all members of the international biology community. It is a place to meet colleagues studying biology and related disciplines, and an arena for hosting colloquia and conferences. The online course in biocomputing, for example, holds its tutorials via BioMOO ('Interactive Online Courses' above).

At BioMOO you can converse, in real time, with anyone else who is currently logged on. The medium for this is your computer keyboard and your Telnet client software. If a group of people arrange to log on to BioMOO at the same time they can hold a meeting just as they would if they had booked a conference venue. The advantage of this method is that colleagues from around the world can attend without having the bother of getting to the location or finding accommodation.

In addition, BioMOO also supports multimedia applications. Thus it is possible to give a presentation, complete with full colour slides and moving images, at a BioMOO conference just as you would at any 'real' conference or meeting. Users who wish to attend such a presentation log on to BioMOO through their Telnet client and then, in parallel, open up a World Wide Web session. Specific instructions on how to do this are detailed in Box 5.2.

Box 5.2 Logging on to BioMOO

1 Using your Telnet client log on to:
   bioinfo.weizmann.ac.il:8888/ To log in as a guest use the form:
   Prompt: guest <name> <password>
   Example: guest rjk testing

2 Resize the Telnet window so that you can see about 5 lines of text. Move this window to the bottom of the screen.

3 Load up your Web browser. Adjust the size of the window so that it sits above your Telnet window. Open the following Web site:
   http://bioinformatics.weizmann.ac.il:8000/

4 When the 'Web authentication form' appears use your BioMOO character name and password if you have a registered character, or the name and password you gave when connecting as a guest.
   Example: Log-in Name: rjk Password: testing

5 Welcome to the BioMOO Lounge.

6 Type 'who' in your Telnet window to see who else is logged on.

Once your log-in has been accepted, you will be presented with a series of hypertext links that allow you to see who else is currently logged in and what objects are available in that room (graphics, files, maps etc.). Figures 5.8 and 5.9 show the BioMOO Lounge and a classroom, and the objects they contain.

To move to another room you simply click on the mouse-sensitive map. To converse with anyone in the room, switch to your Telnet window and type in your question or comment.

Although BioMOO does not require users to wear virtual reality helmets and gloves, it is nevertheless a virtual world. The rooms you meet in exist only as concepts, and although at any point it may feel as if you are conversing with a group of people in one location, in reality the 'delegates' are likely to be scattered throughout the world.

Because MOOs (multiple user dimension object orientated) were originally devised as a computerised version of the adventure game *Dungeons and Dragons*, some people are still reluctant to concede their usefulness in a teaching environment. Any reader who questions the usefulness of BioMOO, however,

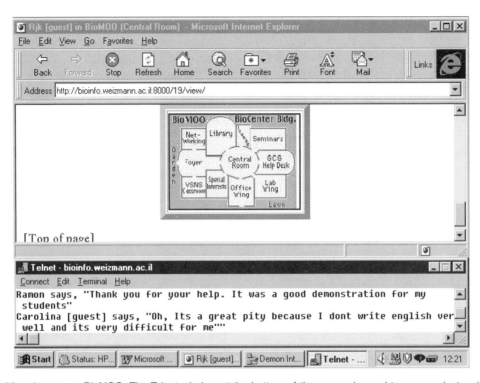

Fig. 5.8 Virtual rooms at BioMOO. The Telnet window at the bottom of the screen is used to communicate with other delegates, whilst the Web window is used to view multimedia applications

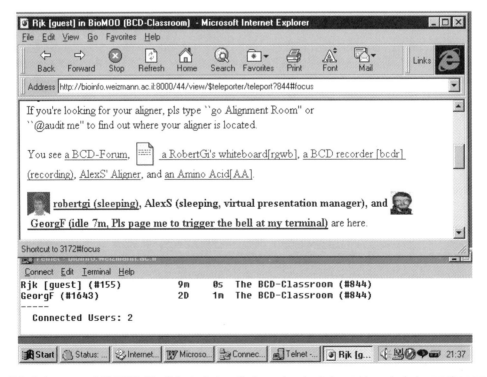

Fig. 5.9 A classroom at BioMOO. The Telnet window displays who else is logged in and what room they are in

should consider where else they could converse with colleagues from around the world in a conference-like environment for the price of a local telephone call.

Medscape Video Conferences

http://www.medscape.com/home/News/
Medscape-News.html#conference

An increasing number of medical conferences – especially those that appeal to a large international audience – broadcast some of the sessions over the Internet. One of the early examples of this occurred in 1996, when live video and sound from the 11th World Congress of Anaesthesiology (WCA) in Sydney, Australia, were broadcast over the Internet using the video conferencing software CU-SeeMe (Fig. 5.10).

CU-SeeMe allows you to see, hear and speak with others, in real time, via the Internet. CU-SeeMe supports both one-to-one and one-to-many video conferencing. To facilitate the latter, the organisation (or person) transmitting the teleconference needs to route

it via a computer running CU-SeeMe reflector software. Computers running this software act as mini television stations. Throughout the Internet-wired world there are a number of public reflectors which, subject to the rules of 'netiquette,' anyone can use.[5]

Perhaps the most exciting thing about CU-SeeMe is that it works over relatively low-speed modem links (28 800 Kbps.) For example, feedback from the 200 virtual delegates of the WCA Conference indicated that the audio reception was 'good' and the video reception 'adequate' to provide a video presence of the speaker.[6] Although the video signal was too weak for the speakers' 35 mm slides to be visualised clearly, there is no reason why in the future the slides could not be hosted on a Web site. Under this scenario virtual delegates would have two browser widows open simultaneously, one for listening to and watching the speaker, and the other for viewing the slide show.

For further details of video conferencing using CU-SeeMe software, and the option to download this client software free of charge, point your Web browser at:

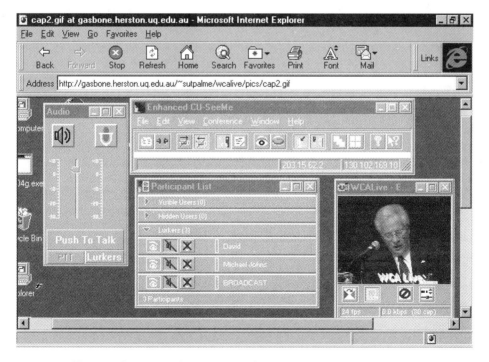

Fig. 5.10 Screen grab from the World Congress of Anaesthesiology, 1996

http://cu-seeme.cornell.edu/#cu-seeme

A different approach to delivering medical conferences over the Internet has been adopted by Medscape. Conscious that health professionals are not always able to attend live conferences – even if they attend as virtual delegates – staff at Medscape record key papers and interviews with the speakers, and then make these available via Real Audio on their Web site. For example, in May 1998 the Medscape site was providing online coverage from the 34th Annual Meeting of the American Society of Clinical Oncology. In addition to being able to access detailed abstracts of the main papers, visitors to this site could listen to a number of speakers discussing their findings (Fig. 5.11).

Real Audio (and Real Video) client software can be downloaded without charge from the RealNetworks Web site at:

http://www.real.com/

Recommended sites for further exploration

Virtual Nurse

http://www.virtualnurse.com/chatlist.html

Health professionals who wish to 'speak' to their peers in real time over the Internet can participate in a growing number of 'chat' forums. Using just the Web browser – with no additional plug-ins – it is possible to communicate with peers from all over the connected world, on virtually any topic.

For nursing staff, one of the more developed services is the Virtual Nurse Web site, which hosts 15 distinct chat rooms. These range from subject-specific rooms such as 'Melissa's Diabetes Room' and the 'HIV Zone Chat', through to rooms aimed at particular communities, such as students (Student chat room) and nurses based in Europe (European Voice of Nursing). Although at times the con-

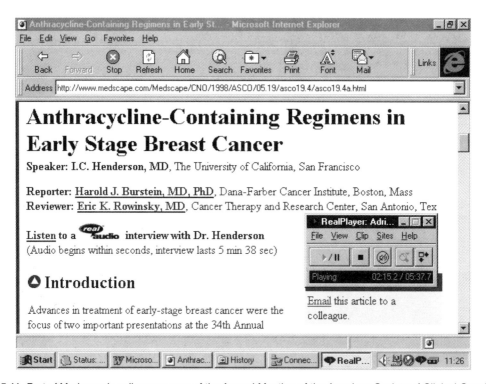

Fig. 5.11 Part of Medscape's online coverage of the Annual Meeting of the American Society of Clinical Oncology

versation can be more social than professional, most rooms advertise times when a particular 'expert' is going to be online, ready to answer questions.

CONCLUSION

As a health sciences librarian one of my responsibilities is to introduce health professionals to the Internet. This is usually done through a hands-on tour of some key medical sites, including many of the ones highlighted in this chapter.

In doing this, the overriding impression I am left with is how much enjoyment they derive from using the Internet. This is not surprising. Indeed, there can be few people who are not attracted by the idea of multimedia textbooks, simulated patient consultations, and meetings conducted in virtual reality.

Apart from making the process of studying and learning more enjoyable, using the Internet as a medium for delivering medical education has other advantages. A study conducted by Sestini,[7] concluded that medical students who had received multimedia training – in conjunction with traditional bedside training – in chest auscultation skills were better able to recognise the correct lung sounds than students who had not. As this chapter has demonstrated, multimedia components are very much to the fore on those Web sites that focus on medical education.

Box 5.3 Using the Internet for medical education: key benefits

- You can study at a time that is convenient to you.
- You do not have to travel to participate in a conference or meeting, but can still enjoy the benefits of live, interactive discussion.
- As virtual meetings attract colleagues and experts from around the world it can be assumed that the discussion will be more informed than that which occurs at a local meeting.
- The delivery of a virtual conference can be done from your own home or place of work, thereby saving time and expense. Funds which would have been consumed on travel and accommodation can now be diverted to patient care.
- A range of state-of-the-art multimedia teaching tools and textbooks is available 24 hours a day, any of which can be easily updated to reflect current knowledge and practice.
- The global nature of the Internet means that resources created by medical institutions around the world can be used to enhance and supplement locally created teaching materials.

Other benefits of using the Internet as a medium for delivering medical education are summarised in Box 5.3.

Although I do not believe the Internet will replace the library or the postgraduate medical centre, it will provide additional opportunities for health professionals to further their medical education. In the longer term this will create a better qualified workforce which, in turn, can deliver patient care more effectively.

REFERENCES

1 Hampton JR 1975 Relative contributions of history-taking, physical examination and laboratory investigation to diagnosis and management of medical outpatients. BMJ 2(5969):486–489
2 Claim made in foreword to the Merck Manual. <URL: http://www.merck.com> [Accessed 27 May 1998]
3 A list of the Royal College's Web sites can be found at: <URL: http://omni.ac.uk/cme/colleges.html> [Accessed 27 May 1998]
4 Branthwaite A 1988 Continuing education for General Practitioners. Royal College of General Practitioners (Occasional Paper, 38)

5 A list of public CU-SeeMe reflectors can be found at: <URL http://www.rocketcharged.com/cu-seeme/general.html> [Accessed 27 May 1998]
6 Palmer TE 1997 WCALive: broadcasting a major medical conference on the Internet. International Journal of Clinical Monitoring and Computing 14(4):209–216
7 Sestini P 1995 Multimedia presentation of lung sounds as a learning aid for medical students. European Respiratory Journal 8(5):783–788

6

E-mail, discussion lists and newsgroups

Box 6.1 Chapter objectives

- Introduce and discuss <u>e-mail</u>, <u>discussion lists</u> and <u>newsgroups</u>, three of the most useful services available on the Internet.

- Explain the function of these, and demonstrate with practical examples their value to health professionals.

- Highlight potential problems and concerns – such as the security of e-mail, or the relevance of newsgroup postings – and suggest ways in which these can be resolved.

INTRODUCTION

For many people, the catalyst for getting connected to the Internet is the wish (or the need) to be able to send and receive electronic mail (e-mail). Indeed, despite the attention that is afforded to applications such as the <u>World Wide Web</u> (and this book is no exception to this) e-mail is still the most widely used service on the Internet.

In addition to being able to communicate with friends and colleagues, e-mail is also the method used for contributing to discussion lists and newsgroups. This chapter looks at these services, and focuses on how they can help health professionals in their day-to-day work. To begin, though, it is necessary to have an understanding of what e-mail is, and why it is so important.

E-MAIL

Defined simply, e-mail is a method for transferring information by electronic means from one location to another. This information can be in the form of a text file or, as is increasingly common, a binary file. Examples of the latter type include wordprocessed documents, spreadsheets or graphics. For completeness it should be noted that e-mail can also be used to retrieve World Wide Web pages and even files from FTP sites.[1]

E-mail: why use it?

To some, it must appear a curious paradox that users of the world's most advanced network of computers – the Internet – rely upon the traditional written word as their main method of communication.

This situation does not reflect some wish to return to bygone days, but rather the realisation that e-mail is the most effective method of communication yet devised. Compared with traditional mail, known by Internet aficionados as 'snail mail', e-mail has many advantages. In particular, for the reasons cited in Box 6.2, it is quick, cheap and efficient.

Compared to the other electronic communications media, telephone and fax, e-mail again scores well. For example, if you wish to communicate with a number of colleagues – some of whom may be overseas – both fax and phone will prove expensive. In addition to this, neither can handle binary files, and the chances of the message reaching the intended recipient will depend on unquantifiable variables such as whether the person is in (to answer the phone), and whether or not the fax machine is engaged, switched on or even loaded with sufficient paper. E-mail messages encounter none of these problems.

Although undoubtedly e-mail is a 'good thing' there is one caveat that should not be overlooked: if you have a dial-up connection to the Internet it is up to *you* to go and collect your mail. Although a message from the other side of the world may hit your mailbox within minutes of it being sent, if you do not routinely empty your mailbox (by dialling into your Internet provider) this significant advantage is lost.

It is also worth pointing out that most Internet providers will only hold mail for a certain period. Demon Internet, for example,

will hold mail for up to 30 days. After this time any mail that has not been collected is returned to the sender. Figure 6.1 illustrates how users who have a dial-up connection to the Internet send and receive e-mail.

E-mail for health professionals

Although the advantages highlighted in Box 6.2 apply to *all* users of e-mail there are other benefits that seem particularly pertinent to health professionals (Box 6.3).

E-mail clients

To be able to compose, send and receive e-mail you must use either a dedicated e-mail client, or have a mail facility within your Web browser. (Both Netscape and the Microsoft Internet Explorer have integrated e-mail capabilities.) Whatever mail client you use it should support the core features identified in Box 6.4.

E-mail to fax

Despite the pervasiveness of the Internet there will still be occasions when you want to com-

---

Box 6.2 The main advantages of e-mail

- **Speed**
  Exactly how long a message takes to get from A to B depends on factors such as network traffic and how many individual networks a particular message has to go through. A survey published in July 1997 reported that 91% of all messages sent by e-mail arrived at their intended destination within 5 minutes of being sent.[2]

- **Cost**
  It costs no more to send a message from London to Australia than it does from London to Oxford. And, although a large file may entail a slightly longer connection to your Internet provider, these costs will be negligible when compared to the cost of air-mailing or sending the same document by courier.

- **Efficiency**
  Assuming you have addressed your message correctly, then for the most part your mail will be delivered. On occasions when this is not possible – the recipient is no longer 'in residence', for example – your mail will be returned. In Internet parlance, mail is 'bounced'.

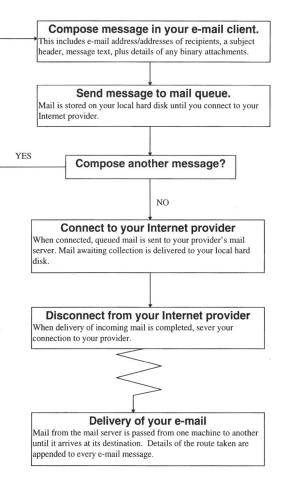

Compose message in your e-mail client.
This includes e-mail address/addresses of recipients, a subject header, message text, plus details of any binary attachments.

Send message to mail queue.
Mail is stored on your local hard disk until you connect to your Internet provider.

YES

Compose another message?

NO

Connect to your Internet provider
When connected, queued mail is sent to your provider's mail server. Mail awaiting collection is delivered to your local hard disk.

Disconnect from your Internet provider
When delivery of incoming mail is completed, sever your connection to your provider.

Delivery of your e-mail
Mail from the mail server is passed from one machine to another until it arrives at its destination. Details of the route taken are appended to every e-mail message.

Fig. 6.1 Sending and receiving e-mail: a schematic overview

Box 6.3 Benefits of e-mail for health professionals

- A scan through the contents of any current medical journal highlights the fact that a great proportion of the articles are co-authored. Using e-mail it is easy to circulate drafts of a paper to all authors, who can comment and add their contribution without ever having to re-key any text.

- If you encounter a rare medical condition and require guidance on how it should be managed you can solicit expert opinion from around the world with just one e-mail message. Further details are given in 'Discussion lists' and 'Newsgroups' (below).

- Because mail is collected at a time that is convenient to you, interruptions to your day can be minimised.

Box 6.4 E-mail software: core requirements

Text editing features
These allow you to cut and paste text.

'Reply' and 'Forward' options
Another factor that has contributed to the popularity of e-mail is the ease with which replies can be generated. On hitting the 'Reply' button, the mail software automatically creates a new message with the addressee details already completed. The original message may also be copied to this file to facilitate the composition of comments and answers. Forwarding mail to other colleagues is achieved by use of the 'Forward' function.

Easy addressing facilities
As e-mail addresses tend to be long and instantly forgettable, it is important that your mail client has an address book function where frequently used e-mail addresses can be stored and accessed. If you have a list of users whom you mail regularly then the option to create a distribution list is also useful.

Ability to attach binary files to your messages
A good mail client will allow you to simply press the 'Attach' button, and prompt you for the name of the file you wish to send. As binary files need to be packaged – encoded – in a particular way before they can be sent over the Internet, a mail client that can do this (and decode received binary files) is to be preferred. Client software that can perform these tasks is said to be MIME compliant.

Support Web addresses
Increasingly, e-mail messages contain references to various Web sites. If your mail software can translate a Web address into a clickable link you can jump directly to that Web page from your e-mail software. Client software that can perform this task is said to be HTTP enabled (Fig. 6.2).

---

municate with someone who only has a fax facility. Using a service devised by The Phone Company, it is now possible to send a fax via e-mail. To use this free service you simply need to address the e-mail message in the following way:

To: **remote-printer.**
firstname_lastname@faxnumber.**iddd.tpc.int**

Replace the fields *firstname* and *lastname* with the name of the person you wish to fax, and *faxnumber* with the appropriate number, prefixed with the appropriate IDDD country code. E-mail attachments (wordprocessed documents, etc.) cannot be sent via this service.

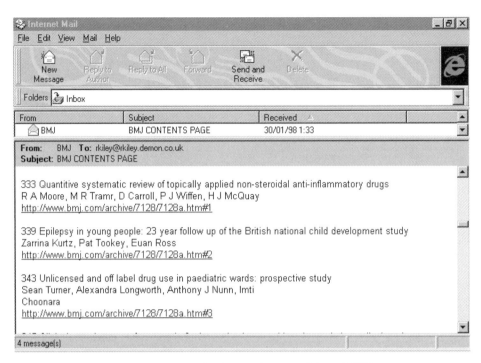

Fig. 6.2 HTTP enabled mail software – hypertext links to WWW pages

An e-mail sent to the following address will arrive as a printed document on my local fax machine:

To: **remote-printer.**
Robert_Kiley@441716118726.**iddd.tpc.int**

The Phone Company is a volunteer organisation that relies on 'local' Internet service providers to host a fax server and provide fax coverage for the local area. At the time of writing, coverage is available in 27 countries, including the United Kingdom, United States and most of Australia. If you wish to check whether the destination you wish to fax to is covered by this scheme, point your browser at:

http://www.tpc.int/verify.html

Free e-mail accounts

Even if you do not have a personal Internet account – perhaps access is enabled via a 'cybercafe' or a public library – you can still have your own e-mail account. Companies such as HotMail and Yahoo! Mail allow any-

one to create their own mail account, free of charge.

Apart from being free, this type of mail account has other useful benefits, as identified in Box 6.5.

For more information and details on how to create a free e-mail account visit either of the following sites:

Box 6.5 Benefits of free Web-based mail accounts

- Using a standard Web browser, e-mail can be collected from any Internet-connected computer anywhere in the world. In contrast, e-mail accounts that form part of the service offered by an ISP can usually only be accessed when you dial into the Internet via that provider. If you are away on business in another country this situation may be inconvenient and expensive.

- As these e-mail services are independent of any ISP your e-mail address will remain the same, irrespective of how many times you change providers or move jobs.

- If you do have multiple mail accounts, you can check all of them through one Web-based e-mail account.

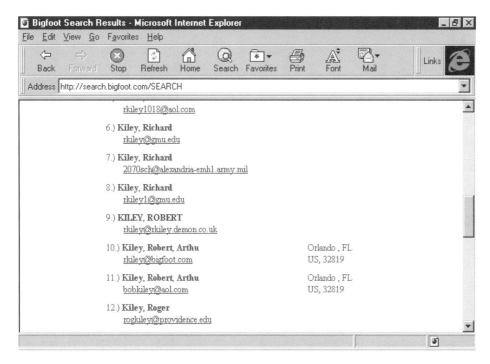

Fig. 6.3 Results of a BigFoot search

HotMail: **http://www.hotmail.com/**
Yahoo! Mail: **http://mail.yahoo.com/**

Finding e-mail addresses

If you dial a telephone number incorrectly you either receive an 'unobtainable' tone or get connected to the wrong person. E-mail addresses work in much the same way, in that incorrectly addressed mail is either 'bounced' (returned to sender) or delivered to a complete stranger. However, whereas telephone users can rely on directory enquiry services to identify the correct number, e-mail users often have to resort to sleuthing and ingenuity.

The easiest way to obtain someone's e-mail address is to telephone them and ask. If this is impractical or inconvenient, however, there are some other methods you can employ.

First, you can use one of the growing number of Internet people-search services, such as BigFoot[3] or Yahoo! People Search.[4] Bigfoot, for example, is a database comprising more than 18 million e-mail addresses, all of which can

be searched by surname and/or Internet domain name. Figure 6.3 shows the results of a Bigfoot search.

In addition to providing e-mail addresses this service also hosts the US 'white pages' listings, collected by Acxiom. Searching this part of the directory enables you to identify the telephone numbers and postal addresses of people resident in the US, along with detailed street maps and driving directions in case you should want to visit the person you are seeking! To search Bigfoot point your browser at:

http://www.bigfoot.com

If a Bigfoot search fails to locate the e-mail address you seek, a second approach is to search the Mailbase membership database (see below). Although only 130 000 e-mail addresses are stored here, the education and research focus of the Mailbase discussion lists means that the find rate for health professionals is relatively high.

To search this index point your Web browser at:

http://www.mailbase.ac.uk/search.html

Finally, if you know *where* the person you are seeking is employed, you can run a search to see if the employing institution has a presence on the World Wide Web. (These pages can be found through a Web search engine, as discussed in Chapter 3.) If it has a presence, then it is possible that the Web site will have a link to a staff index that can either be searched or browsed.

Security

Mail sent electronically is often likened to a postcard, in that it can be read as it makes its way from sender to recipient. However, whereas a postman or sorting clerk will tire long before he reads anything he can use to his advantage, computer programs looking for 'trigger terms' – such as credit card numbers – never will. Consequently, if you are going to use e-mail to send sensitive or confidential data, encryption is highly recommended.

In essence there are two kinds of encrypting techniques. The first, made available by some mail clients, enables you to transform your mail into a random string of characters which can only be deciphered if the recipient knows the password. As sending the password by e-mail would negate the object of the exercise, the sender must find some other way of notifying the recipient of the correct password. As you can imagine, this is not particularly practical and thus not widely used.

A second and better method is based on public/private key encryption. Users of this technique employ a piece of software to generate two alphanumeric 'keys'. The private key, held on the user's computer, is never disclosed, but the public key is made available to everyone. Anyone can then use this public key to send an encrypted message to this person, but *only* the recipient, who has the second half of the key, can decrypt the message.

If you wish to use this form of encryption, a freeware program known as Pretty Good Privacy (PGP) can be freely downloaded from either of the following locations:

Non-US residents: **http://www.pgpi.com/**
US residents: **http://mit.edu/network/pgp.html**

The reason that there are two sites is that it is illegal to export (or download) this software from the United States. The US State Department considers PGP to be strong cryptographic technology and, as such, regulates its export via the International Traffic in Arms Regulations (ITAR). It should be made clear, however, that as long as you download PGP from the appropriate location, it is perfectly legal to use.

The attempt by the US government to stop this technology falling into 'enemy' hands reflects the fact that it is virtually impossible to decipher PGP-encrypted mail.

Viruses

Over the past 18 months or so there has been much talk in the press about computer viruses being transmitted by e-mail.[5] The most famous – and worrying – of these has been the 'Winword.concept' macro virus, which attaches itself to documents created with Microsoft's Word for Windows. When the recipient opens a mail item infected with this virus, a macro – a set of predefined keystrokes – is executed, with potentially disastrous results. Although in its original form the virus did no damage – it merely contained the comment 'that's enough to prove my point' – creating a macro that could delete files is perfectly possible.

Although initially describing this virus as little more than a 'prank', widespread concern about the potential of this macro has forced Microsoft to revise its attitude. Users of Microsoft Word are now advised that a 'scanning tool must be installed by anyone who opens files that are received through e-mail, or downloaded from the Internet'. For more information about macro viruses and software tools to help thwart them, point your browser at:

http://www.microsoft.com/office/antivirus/

To keep this threat in proportion, one should remember that most messages received electronically are text files and as such must be virus-free. When a file is accompanied with a binary attachment, it is always good practice to scan it with an up-to-date virus checker before it is opened.

Conventions and netiquette

When conversing by telephone, our tone of voice adds meaning to what we are saying. Similarly, when sending a letter by post we clarify the message in a variety of ways: job applications tend to be submitted on high-quality vellum-like paper, whilst letters to a lover may be enclosed in a scented envelope, adorned with the acronym SWALK. The recipient of a message sent electronically, however, has to rely *exclusively* on the written word.

To minimise the risk of misunderstandings, e-mail users have devised various codes (knows as smiley's or emote-icons) that you can add to the text to clarify your meaning. For example, to indicate that you are joking you can append your comments with a :-) (tilt your head through 90° to see this more clearly). Should you ever wish to indicate that you are a drunk, devilish chef with a toupee, a moustache and double chin, use the following:

C=}>;*())

For more examples of this art ;-), see the Smiley's Server at:

http://www.pop.at/smileys

A good rule of thumb, however, is that if your message is likely to be misunderstood, rephrase it.

To minimise the amount of text you have to type and to keep messages concise, a number of e-mail acronyms have been adopted. IM(H)O 'in my (humble) opinion', BTW 'by the way' and TIA 'thanks in advance' are perhaps the most common and most useful.

Finally, good netiquette (etiquette on the Internet) dictates that:

• your messages should not be composed in CAPITAL LETTERS – it appears as if you are shouting;
• your e-mail signature should be no more than three lines long ;
• mailings to a newsgroup or discussion list (see below) should be relevant and worthwhile. Reposting someone else's

message with the comment 'I agree' will not endear you to other Internet users.

ELECTRONIC DISCUSSION LISTS

Discussion lists (or mailing lists as they are sometimes called), are subject-specific discussion groups that are participated in and distributed by e-mail. Once a user has joined a list – research into drug abuse or medical informatics, for example – every message that is subsequently posted to that list is copied to the individual's electronic mailbox. This task is performed by computer programs known as listservers.

Discussion lists are an excellent way in which health professionals can seek opinions, air concerns and discuss topics of mutual interest. For example, subscribers to the *evidence-based-health*[6] mailing list have, in the past few weeks, discussed the use of EBM in primary care clinics, discussed the efficacy of Ticlopidine for secondary prevention of stroke, and have been kept informed of relevant courses and conferences (Fig. 6.4).

It should be noted, however, that the *majority* of discussion lists are open to everyone. Although the discussion list *gp-uk*[7] – with its emphasis on education and training for general practitioners in the United Kingdom – will be of little interest to most people, there is nothing to stop *anyone* following the discussions or posting questions to the list.

In recognition of this, a number of moderated medical discussion lists have started to appear. For example, potential subscribers to *SURGINET*[8] – a forum for the discussion of all aspects of general surgery – have to demonstrate that they are medically qualified *before* they are admitted to the list. Although this means that someone has to manually vet potential subscribers, the end result should be a more informed, and thus more useful, discussion group.

Whatever the status of the list, however, all subscribers should remember how easy it is to forward e-mail to other people. A message you thought was going to a select and discreet group of people can be forwarded, at the touch of a button, to other lists and other people.

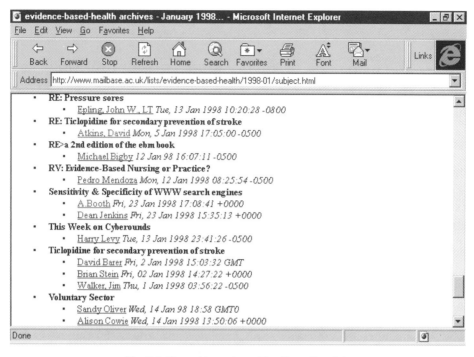

Fig. 6.4 The evidence-based health mailing list

With this in mind you should never send anything by e-mail that you would not want to become public knowledge.

Finding lists pertinent to your interests

If you total the number of mailing lists hosted by the four major listservers (Listserv, Listprocessor, Majordomo and Mailbase) you will discover that you have the option to subscribe to more than 85 000 discussion lists.

To identify which lists most closely match your interests, either consult one of the medical indexing resources, such as Medical Matrix or OMNI (Ch. 3), or search the listserver database at the following address:

http://www.liszt.com/

As an example of the range of lists available, a search for 'arthritis' identified five potentially relevant discussion forums, including *arthritis-l*, a general discussion forum about arthritis, and *OMERACT*, a tightly defined list that looks exclusively at outcome measures in rheumatoid arthritis clinical trials.

The Liszt database also provides additional information about each list, including the average number of postings and whether the list is open or closed. If this information is unavailable, instruction is provided on how to obtain this data.

Although the coverage of the Liszt database is extensive it does not index the 1800+ discussion lists hosted by Mailbase. As these lists originate in the UK and are only established if they can be seen to benefit higher education and research communities, they are particularly useful to health professionals practising in the UK. Names and descriptions of Mailbase lists can be searched at:

http://www.mailbase.ac.uk/search.html

The Mailbase server also maintains an archive of all discussion list postings. Users can access this resource to assess the quality and relevance of a discussion list *before* subscribing. The fact that mailings are archived further reinforces the need to be circumspect when participating in a group discussions.[9]

Joining, contributing and leaving a discussion list

To join a discussion list you simply send an e-mail to the listserver that hosts the list, indicating the name of the list you wish to subscribe to and your 'real' name. There is no need to include your e-mail address, as this will be picked up automatically by the listserver. Figure 6.5 shows how you would join the list *gp-uk*.

An automatic acknowledgement of your subscription will be mailed to you, along with instructions on how to contribute to the list and how to leave it.

It may sound somewhat trivial and pedantic, but perhaps the most important thing to learn about discussion lists is the difference between the address of the *mailing list* and the address of the *listserver*. All e-mail relating to the administration of the list (subscribing, suspending etc.) must be sent to the listserver, whereas contributions to the discussion are sent to the list.

Once you have joined a discussion list it is important to collect your e-mail on a regular basis. Contributing to a discussion that took place some time ago and has now moved on will not endear you to the other list members.

You should also be aware that some discussion lists are very active. The *gp-uk* list, for example, receives on average 555 messages every month. If you defer collecting your mail for a few days you may be surprised by the number of messages that have accumulated, and how long it takes to download and read them.

Similarly, if you are going to be away for a long time, check the documentation that was mailed with your subscription confirmation to see if the listserver supports 'suspend' and 'resume' functions.

Finally, netiquette and common sense dictate that all contributions should be relevant, and, unless specifically permitted, you should not use a discussion list for advertising purposes.

To:	mailbase@mailbase.ac.uk
Subject: *Leave blank*	
Text:	subscribe gp-uk *firstname surname*

Fig. 6.5 Joining the list *gp-uk*: Note that this e-mail is sent to the listserver for this group

USENET NEWS – NEWSGROUPS

Newsgroups are another way in which the Internet facilitates group communication. Arranged on a subject-specific basis, newsgroups enable groups of like-minded people to ask questions, raise concerns and discuss topics of mutual interest. For example, people who are interested in political economics in the UK can read and contribute to the *uk.politics.economics* newsgroup, whilst aficionados of lotteries may find the *rec.gambling.lottery* newsgroup essential reading. Alternatively, health professionals with a special interest in cardiology or AIDS may care to follow the discussions in the *sci.med.cardiology* or *sci.med.aids* newsgroups.

Current estimates suggest that there are over 50 000 newsgroups, catering for every interest, specialty and perversion known to man. The tabloid-generated myth that the Internet is merely a repository of pornography is, to a large degree, the consequence of a small minority of Internet newsgroups.

Although the purpose of newsgroups and discussion lists is the same – that is, to share information on a groupwide basis – they differ in the following respects:

- Postings to a newsgroup are held on a Newsgroup server; they are *not* copied to your personal electronic mailbox.
- You do not formally subscribe to a newsgroup.

Not subscribing means that if, on a particular day, you wish to read postings made to the *sci.med.diseases.hepatitis* newsgroup you merely indicate this via your newsgroup client (see below). There is no newsgroup equivalent of the listserver.

Internet newsgroups attract huge international audiences, and as such are excellent ways to solicit opinions and seek advice. For example, the newsgroup *news.newusers.questions*, set up as a question and answer forum for users new to Usenet, attracts a daily readership of 160 000 people.[10] Although the more specialised groups attract smaller audiences, they are still fairly substantial. The *sci.med.aids* newsgroup attracts 26 000 readers, and even the highly specific *sci.med.telemedicine* newsgroup boasts a daily readership of around 14 000.[11]

To participate in this global distributed discussion system you must have the facilities outlined in Box 6.6.

The choice of newsreader client will depend upon your operating system and what is currently available. Whichever client you opt for, though, it should support:

- message 'threading' (Fig. 6.6)
- an offline reading facility.

Message threading sorts messages by the heading, so that replies are shown next to the original message. Offline reading allows you

---

Box 6.6 Newsgroups: requirements for participation

- Your Internet provider must offer a 'newsfeed' service. Messages sent to newsgroups are propagated around the Internet by a protocol known as NNTP (network news transport protocol). If your provider does not have a NNTP server you can use a public news server such as the WReN (Web Reading News) interface, hosted by Supernews. See: **http://wren.supernews.com/**

- You must have a client on your computer that can interpret data sent from a NNTP server. Typically, this will take the form of a dedicated newsreader, or your Web browser if it has been 'news enabled' (Appendix B).

---

to collect your messages from the NNTP server but read them once your connection to your Internet provider has been severed.

Arrangement of newsgroups

To help the user navigate his way through the mass of newsgroups, a hierarchical approach has been adopted. Table 6.1 shows the most important newsgroup categories, with exam-

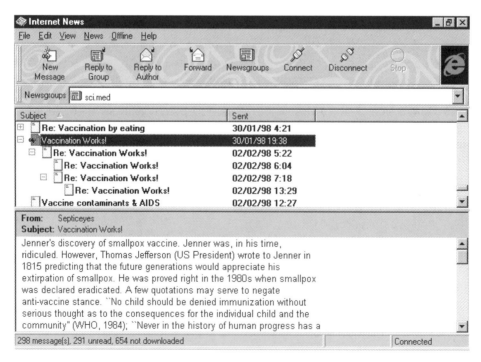

Fig. 6.6 Message threading

Table 6.1 Newsgroup hierarchy

Category	Topic	Example
alt	Alternative	alt.comics.batman
bionet	Biology	bionet.genone.gene-structure
comp	Computers	comp.software.year-2000
misc	Miscellaneous	misc.jobs.offered
news	Topics on Usenet newsgroups	news.newusers.questions
rec	Recreational	rec.collecting.stamps
sci	Sciences	sci.med.aids
soc	Society – cultural	soc.history.war.world-war-ii
talk	Talk	talk.politics.medicine

ples to illustrate how the top-level category is further subdivided.

In addition to these category groups, you may also encounter newsgroups that are restricted to specific regions or organisations. Subscribers to Demon Internet, for example, have access to a range of *demon* newsgroups where problems, questions and news specific to Demon users can be discussed.

Precisely which newsgroups are available will be determined by your Internet provider. However, although some will not have a news-feed to the *alt.sex* range of newsgroups, the majority of providers can be expected to carry the scientific range of newsgroups most sought after by health professionals.

Finding relevant newsgroups

With so many newsgroups available, identifying relevant ones can be a time-consuming process. Indeed, even if your newsreader client supports keyword searching of newsgroup titles, relevant groups may still be overlooked. A title search for a newsgroup on prostatic hypertrophy, for example, would not identify the group *sci.med.prostate.bph* (bph is an acronym for benign prostatic hypertrophy).

This problem, however, has been addressed by the DejaNews Interest Finder, which identifies relevant newsgroups by comparing your interests with articles in the DejaNews archive. For example, a search for the phrase 'aortic stenosis' indicates that the *sci.med.cardiology* newsgroup best caters for this specialty, whilst

professionals interested in 'osteoporosis' could read the *alt.support.menopause sci.med.diseases.osteoporosis* and *sci.med.nutrition* newsgroups (Fig. 6.7). The DejaNews Interest Finder can be accessed at:

http://www.dejanews.com/home_if.shtml

Filtering the news

Although newsgroups can be interesting, informative and entertaining, they are also very time-consuming. A typical newsgroup in the *sci.med* hierarchy will generate around 20 postings a day. Although this number is manageable, if you subscribe to other equally active newsgroups and/or forget to collect the news on a particular day, it is not long before information overload is experienced.

In addition to this issue of quantity there is also the problem of relevance. For example, if you are interested in following and participating in discussions on breast cancer it would appear to make sense to subscribe to groups such as *sci.med.diseases.cancer* and *sci.med.pathology*. However, as both groups cover a fairly broad spectrum it is probable that most of the discussion will *not* be focused on this specialty.

As if this scenario were not bad enough, there is the related problem that *other* newsgroups may also carry postings on breast cancer. A search on the DejaNews database indicates that the groups *sci.med*, *sci.environment*, *bionet.general* and *sci.psychology.misc* regularly carry postings on this topic.

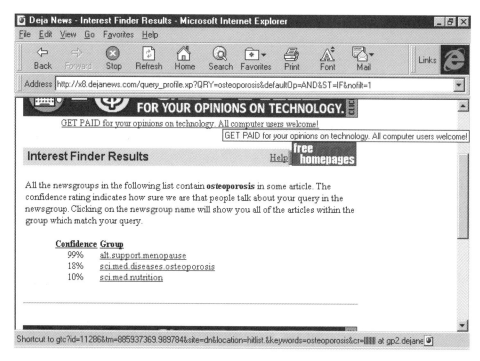

Fig. 6.7 DejaNews interest finder

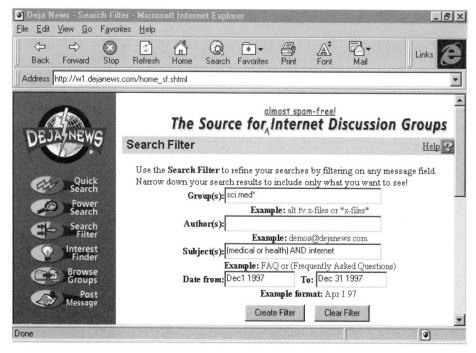

Fig. 6.8 DejaNews search filter

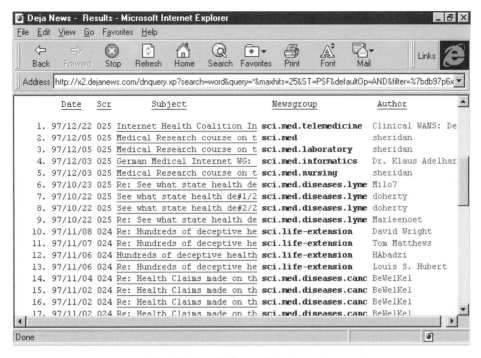

Fig. 6.9 Results from a filtered search

One solution to this is to define a search filter, which you can run against the DejaNews database. This filter can specify which newsgroups should be scanned, what keywords you wish to search for, and what period of time the search should cover. Figures 6.8 and 6.9 show the search filter (and the results) established to monitor postings to the *sci.med.* hierarchy of newsgroups on the subject medical information on the Internet. To find *new* postings I simply change the date field.

CONCLUSION

A recent article in the *Canadian Medical Association Journal*[12] drew attention to the fact that psychiatrists at the University of Michigan are counselling patients via e-mail. An earlier article in the *BMJ* highlighted the emerging practice of patients using e-mail to communicate with health professionals.[13] Leaving aside issues such as whether this medium is appropriate for sensitive and confidential data, this highlights the fact that e-mail

has become an accepted and popular mode of communication.

In addition to facilitating the doctor/patient relationship, studies also show that doctor/doctor relationships are enhanced by e-mail. A study by Singarella et al,[14] found that doctors working in two health sciences institutions used e-mail in preference to the telephone or the traditional letter. With e-mail, response rates were deemed to be quicker and communication errors reduced.

This chapter has demonstrated how e-mail is used to communicate on a groupwide basis through discussion lists and newsgroups. Despite the obvious benefits these can deliver to health professionals, it is important to remember that the quality of information posted in these forums is highly variable. Indeed, a study conducted by Desai et al[15] concluded that 20% of all postings to the *sci.med.pharmacy* newsgroup contained information that independent experts classified as harmful. In the light of this, I suspect that there will be an increasing tendency to establish physician-only discussion lists, where the relevance of the questions and the quality of the answers can be assured.

It should also be emphasised that in this litigation-minded world, newsgroup or discussion list postings that request help in diagnosing or treating a particular medical condition should be ignored, or answered with disclaimers that would render future legal action futile.

Having drawn attention to these concerns, I would still urge all health professionals to participate in Internet-based group discussions. Provided you select your lists and newsgroups with care, you will find them informative, interesting and enjoyable.

REFERENCES

1 Although such services are of use to people who have a 'mail-only' Internet connection, as the rest of this book has assumed that you have a full Internet connection, with a World Wide Web browser, I am not going to detail how these tasks can be performed by e-mail. If you require this information then obtain a copy of Bob Rankin's *Guide to Offline Internet Access* by sending the following message:

> To: mailbase@mailbase.ac.uk
> Subject: *Leave blank*
> Text: send lis-iis e-access-inet.txt

If your mailer automatically appends a signature to your mail, disable this function for this message.

2 Inverse Network Technology **<URL: http://www.inversenet.com/news/ pr_07-22-97>** [Accessed 23 January 1998]

3 Bigfoot: **<URL:http://www.bigfoot.com/>** [Accessed 23 January 1998]

4 Yahoo! People Search: **<URL: http:// www.yahoo.co.uk/mailsearch/email.html>** [Accessed 2 February 1998]

5 Stone D 1996 The WinWord.concept virus. PC Magazine, 6 February. **<URL: http:// www.zdnet.com/pcmag/issues/1503/pcm00100.htm>** [Accessed 18 January 1998]

6 *evidence-based-health* is a Mailbase discussion list. To subscribe send the following message:

> To: mailbase@mailbase.ac.uk
> Subject: *Blank*
> Text: Subscribe evidence-based-health
>   *firstname surname*

7 *gp-uk* is a Mailbase discussion list. To subscribe send the following message:

> To: mailbase@mailbase.ac.uk
> Subject: *Blank*
> Text: Subscribe gp-uk *firstname surname*

8 Before you can join the Surginet discussion list you need to demonstrate your medical credentials. Contact: Tom Gilas at: tgilas@hookup.net

9 Mailbase Lists **<URL: http://www.mailbase.ac.uk/ lists.html>** [Accessed 22 July 1998]

10 Tile.Net **<URL: http://www.tile.net/news/ newsnewu.html>**[Accessed 22 July 1998]

11 Tile.Net **<URL: http://tile.net/news/scimedaids.html>** [Accessed 24 January 1998] Tile.Net **<URL: http:// tile.net/news/scimedtelemedicine.html>** [Accessed 24 January 1998]

12 Johnston C 1996 Psychiatrist says counselling via e-mail may be yet another medical use for Internet. Canadian Medical Association Journal 155(11): 1606–1607

13 Sellu D 1996 Clinical encounters in cyberspace. BMJ 312(7022):49

14 Singarella T, Baxter J, Sandefur RR, Emery CC 1993 The effects of electronic mail on communication in two health sciences institutions. Journal of Medical Systems 17(2):69–86

15 Desai NS, Dole EJ, Yeatman ST, Troutman WG 1997 Evaluation of drug information in an Internet newsgroup. Journal of the American Pharmaceutical Association NS34(4):391–394

7

The quality issue

Box 7.1 Chapter objectives

- Highlight some of the dubious health claims that can be found on the Internet.
- Provide guidelines to help you evaluate the information you find on the Internet.
- Discuss a number of initiatives that are being developed to counter the problem of medical misinformation.

INTRODUCTION

A search of the medical literature over the past 18 months highlights a growing concern about the quality of health information that can be found on the Internet.[1–8] Claims that sea cucumber can be 'effective in the treatment of osteoarthritis'[9] or that 'aloe vera can cure AIDS'[10] are just two examples of the dubious claims that litter the Internet (Fig. 7.1). Recently, in an attempt to alert consumers to this growing phenomenon, the Federal Trade Commission published a statement warning all Internet users to be 'wary of unscrupulous marketers who use cyberspace to peddle "miracle" treatments and cures'.[11]

The purpose of this chapter is to examine some of the more dubious health claims that are evident on the Internet and, more importantly, provide guidelines that will help you appraise the quality of the information you find.

QUACKERY ON THE WEB

Stories that the Internet is being used to market miracle cures should come as no surprise.

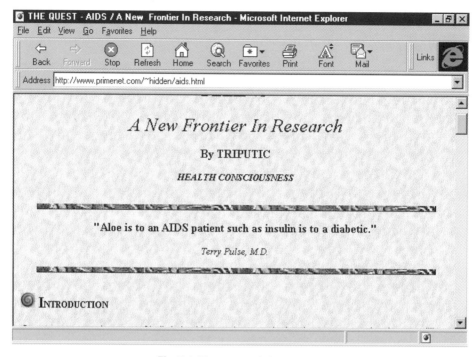

Fig. 7.1 The power of aloe vera?

The market, and the potential profit for 'cure-all remedies' is huge, whilst the cost of setting up a credible-looking Web site is virtually nothing. Indeed, most Internet service providers give their customers Web space as part of their annual subscription fee. Although such Web sites are usually identifiable in the URL – my personal Web pages, for example, are at **http://www.rkiley.demon.co.uk** – for a nominal fee this can be changed to a more plausible-sounding address. Anyone who wished to peddle a 'cure' for baldness might consider that buying a domain name, such as **http://www.alopecia.org**, might give their Web page an aura of authenticity and authority, and thus increase sales.

Although examples of medical misinformation on the Internet are numerous, analysis shows that they all fit within one of the following distinct groups:

- Web sites that contain **cure-all remedies** – based on scant or no medical evidence.
- Web sites that contain **inaccurate information** – although recognising that much of the information in this category has been posted in good faith.
- Web sites which contain **biased information** – usually as a result of pharmaceutical sponsorship.

Cure-all remedies

The ease with which 'cure-all remedies' can be found on the Internet can best be demonstrated by example: a search on the AltaVista search engine for Web sites that discussed 'cancer cure' identified a staggering 1273 documents. Within the first five hits of this search the Royal Rife Research Society Web page, 'The Cancer Cure that Worked',[12] was identified (Fig. 7.2).

The Royal Rife Research Society (RRRS), founded in honour of Royal Raymond Rife, 'one of the greatest scientific geniuses of the 20th century', promotes the notion that all types of cancer can be cured by use of a special frequency instrument. In 1932, so the RRRS claims, Rife discovered that every disease has

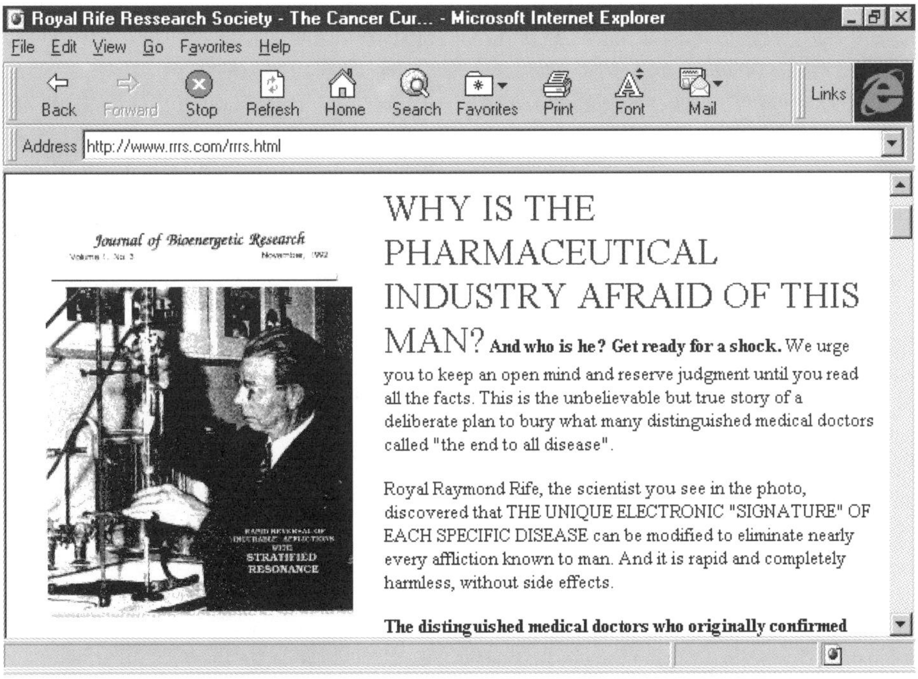

Fig. 7.2 Royal Rife Research Society – the cancer cure that worked

its own 'unique electronic signature' which, once identified, can be modified to 'eliminate nearly every affliction known to man'. With such extravagant claims being made it is not surprising to learn that the frequency instrument is also 'easy to use, quick, and completely harmless'.

The RRRS also claims that the University of Southern California sponsored research into this electronic therapy on the terminally ill, with amazing results: 'after 130 days, every patient in the study had recovered without side effects of any kind'. In true conspiracy theorist style, the RRRS claims that this information is being deliberately withheld from the public by the pharmaceutical industry, which fears it would be put out of business if information about the frequency instrument became widely known. Although the RRRS site states that it does not manufacture, sell, repair or have parts for this instrument, if you e-mail them your postal address they will inform you where it can be purchased.

A search of both the MEDLINE (1966–April 1998) and CancerLit databases finds no refer-

ence to this type of cancer treatment. Moreover, on contacting the Norris Cancer Center at the University of Southern California (USC) to see if they knew of the research they had allegedly sponsored, I received a reply from the Executive Director of the USC Health Sciences Division informing me that:

> 'We have been looking into the claim made by the RRRS and so far have found nothing even remotely related to substantiate it.' (Brenda Maceo, [maceo@hsc.usc.edu] personal communication, 1998).[13]

Another 'cancer cure' that is receiving a lot of coverage on the Internet is shark cartilage. The Shark Cartilage Tumor Inhibitor Web site,[14] for example, gives details of a study conducted by Dr Roscoe L. Van Zandt which showed that in women with advanced breast tumours a daily dose of orally administered shark cartilage had a significant impact on reducing tumour size:

> 'After six weeks all the tumours had significantly reduced in size! In three cases the tumours

had become encapsulated. In two cases in which the tumours had become attached to the chest wall, they became detached and free floating. Also, two women experienced disappearance of their uterine fibroid tumours!'

These findings, along with an order form to purchase shark cartilage, can still be found on this Web site despite the fact that in May 1997, at the American Society of Clinical Oncology's annual meeting, rigorous research was presented which concluded, 'shark cartilage was inactive in patients with advanced stage cancer and specifically in patients with breast, colon, lung and prostate cancer'.[15]

Other unproven and potentially harmful medical products available for purchase over the Internet include a do-it-yourself abortion and sterilisation kit. The FDA, which conducted a health hazard assessment of this product, concluded that using this kit without the supervision of a physician 'could cause heavy vaginal bleeding and even death'.[16]

The FDA is also investigating a resurgence of abuse of the drug gammahydroxybutyrate (GHB), known colloquially as the date-rape drug. GHB, described by its supporters as a 'life enhancing, fat reducing, muscle building, prosexual, and potentially life extending drug', is unapproved in the US and controlled by the Medicines Act in the UK. A recent statement by the FDA alerted consumers to the dangers of this product with the warning that 'a number of deaths have been linked to the consumption of GHB product'.[17] Despite this, anyone with access to the Internet can visit the GHBInfo Web site[18] and obtain this product. By exploiting a legal loophole, the Centurion Aging Research Laboratory – which runs the GHBInfo Web site – sells the chemical components in kit form, with instructions on how they can be combined to produce GHB.

Inaccurate medical information

Not all medical quackery that appears on the Internet, however, has a commercial – get-rich-quick – agenda. There are numerous Web sites where individual users and organisations post

information in good faith, oblivious of the fact that it is inaccurate or misleading.

In 1997, the *BMJ* published a study conducted by Impicciatore[4] which demonstrated the dangers of using the Internet to find information about how a parent should manage a child with fever. Looking at 41 Web sites where this topic was discussed, only four (10%) adhered closely to published recommendations. Thus, whereas the agreed protocol states that a feverish child should be sponged using tepid water, and only after paracetamol has been administered, a mere 15% of the selected Web sites advised this. More worrying was the finding that two of the sites recommended cold sponging, or sponging with alcohol: cold sponging leads to shivering, which serves to raise the body temperature, whilst inhalation of alcohol may induce hypoglycaemia and coma in children.[19]

Medical misinformation is not, however, restricted to the World Wide Web. A study conducted by Culver[20] found that 90% of the messages sent to the discussion list SOREHAND – a list dedicated to the discussion of painful hand and arm conditions – were authored by persons *without* medical training.

This situation is also evident in the disease-support Usenet newsgroups. Figure 7.3 shows a number of postings that were sent to the *alt.support.cancer.prostate* newsgroup on the topic of whether radiation therapy is more effective than surgery in managing cancer of the prostate. What is significant is that in this random selection *all* the information offered was based on personal and anecdotal experience: not a single reply contained any citation to published studies that supported their own experiences.

The dangers of unsupported testimonies become even greater when specific medications are under debate. A recent discussion in the *alt.support.headaches.migraine* newsgroup focused on the efficacy, or otherwise, of imitrex, verapamil and naproxen. As would be expected, there were advocates for and against each drug, but again not a single posting cited any supporting evidence-based medical research.

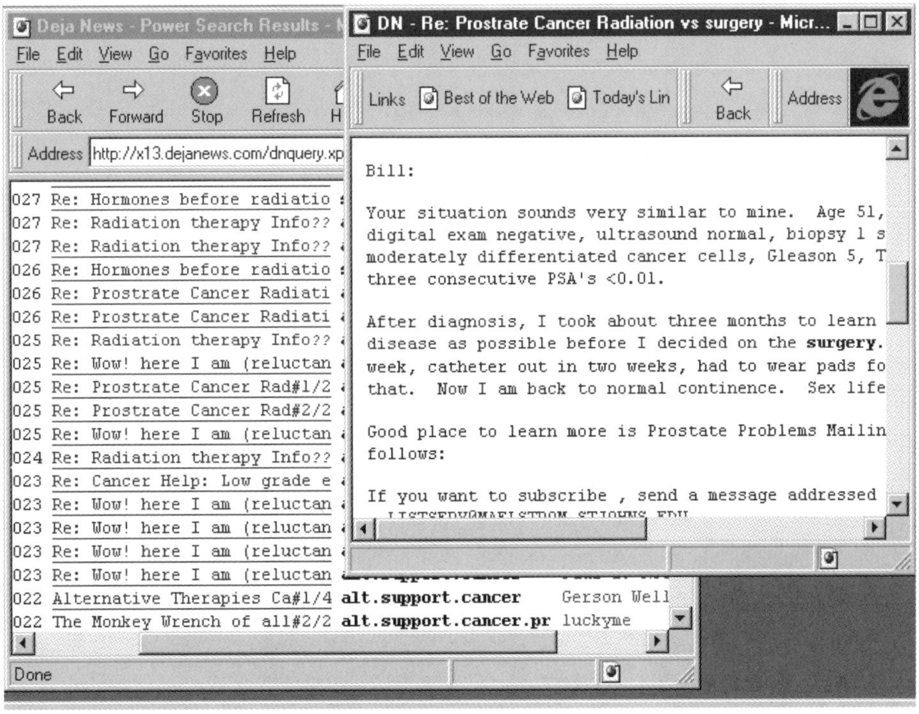

Fig. 7.3 Unsupported testimonies sent to the *alt.support.cancer.prostate* newsgroup

Biased information

When an article is accepted for publication in a peer-reviewed medical journal such as the *Lancet* or *JAMA*, authors have to comply with the guidelines set out by the Vancouver Group. Prominent among these is the requirement that the author disclose any sponsorship or conflict of interest, and whether or not the 'supporting agency controlled or influenced the decision to submit the final manuscript for publication'.

Out on the Internet, however, rules are not so easy to define and even harder to police. Inevitably, therefore, some of the medical information you may find on the Internet may not be as independent and free of bias as you imagine.

One of the best examples of subtle pharmaceutical advertising I have come across is the Café Herpes Web site. Designed to look like an online café, with menus and waiters, the site has a 'reading lounge' where you can learn about genital herpes, a 'terrace' which pro-

vides links to online support groups and related Web sites, and an 'Espresso bar' where 'double servings of product information' await you (Fig. 7.4).

This site, however, is entirely owned by the drug manufacturer SmithKline-Beecham. Although this fact *is* displayed on the Café Herpes Home Page, it is not disclosed in the Espresso Bar page, where the drug Famvir – manufactured by SmithKline Beecham – is recommended for the treatment and suppression of recurrent genital herpes (Fig. 7.5).

It is also possible for companies and organisations to rent advertising space at popular Web sites and get their advertisements displayed when trigger keywords are used. At the time of writing, a search for 'cancer' at the Yahoo! site brings up a banner advertisement for Mediconsult, the consumer health marketing company (Fig. 7.6). Similarly, when searching the Medscape drugs databank[22] an advertisement for Biaxin clarithromycin tablets appears. Clicking on the banner takes you to

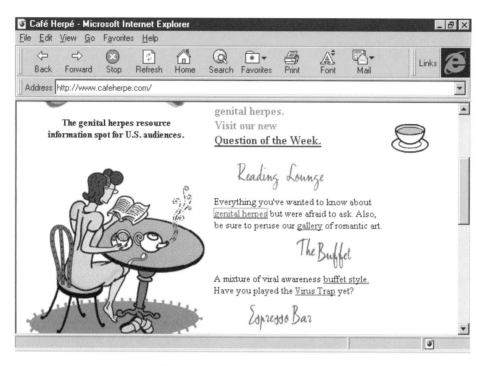

Fig. 7.4 The Café Herpes Web site

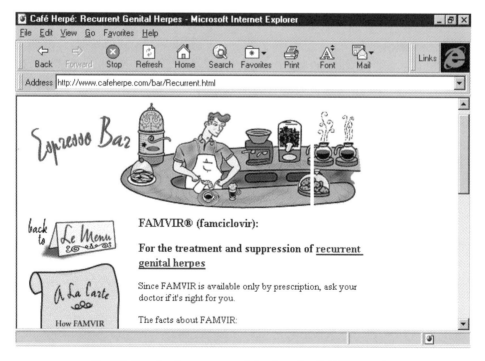

Fig. 7.5 Famvir – the recommendation from the Café Herpes site

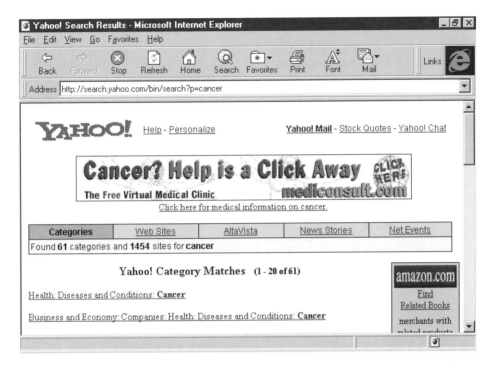

Fig. 7.6 Trigger advertising at Yahoo!. A search for cancer triggers an advertisement for MediConsult

the Abbott Laboratories – who manufacture this drug – Web site, where full prescribing information is available.

In the examples cited here I am *not* questioning the authority of the information provided by the relevant drug companies, but merely pointing out how easy it is to stumble across medical information which, by definition, has an intrinsic bias.

EVALUATING MEDICAL INFORMATION

Although, as has been demonstrated, it is fairly easy to find information which may not be of the desired quality, it is also reasonably easy to apply some basic critical appraisal techniques to weed the information you retrieve.

Based on the work undertaken by Silberg,[5] the principles set out in Box 7.2 provide a means by which accountability can be determined. Any medical Web page that fails to comply with these minimum standards should be rejected.

QUALITY INITIATIVES

Increased awareness of the problems relating to the quality of medical information on the Internet have spurred a number of individuals and organisations to devise new ways of helping Internet users find medical resources that meet a defined quality threshold. These initia-

---

Box 7.2 Evaluating Web pages

- **Authorship**
  The author(s) of a Web page, along with their affiliations and credentials, should be clearly stated. Ideally, there should be the facility to contact the author(s) by e-mail.

- **Attribution**
  If a Web site is quoting research or evidence then the source of this data must be explicitly stated.

- **Disclosure**
  The owner of the Web site must be prominently displayed, along with any sponsorship or advertising deals that could constitute a potential conflict of interest.

- **Currency**
  Web pages should indicate when the page was created, and when it was last updated.

tives fall into one of three categories, each of which is discussed below:

- Initiatives which give **badges of approval** to sites that meet the defined quality criteria.
- Initiatives which provide the user with a **rating tool** to assess the quality of any Web site.
- Initiatives that use **Web technology to filter** medical information.

Badges of approval

Awards such as the 'Infoseek Cool Site', 'NetGuide's Platinum Site', '5 Star Site' and 'MDLink Approved' seem to appear on virtually every Web site. Indeed, it is becoming increasingly difficult to find a Web site that does *not* boast some award. The excellent OncoLink site (Ch. 4) currently displays 40 award badges!

Despite being designed to help the Internet surfer identify the good site from the bad, the fact that badges of approval tend to be based on characteristics such as Web design, innova-

tion and freshness – rather than the quality of the information – means they are inappropriate for assessing medical Web sites. One badge, however, that *does* indicate that the medical information is of a defined standard is the Health on the Net Foundation logo (Fig. 7.7).

The Health on the Net Foundation has devised an eight-point *Code of Conduct* for medical Web sites, central to which is the principle that medical information must 'only be given by medically trained and qualified professionals'. When this condition cannot be met there must be a 'clear statement …that a piece of advice offered is from a non-medically qualified individual'.

Web sites that comply with the code are granted the right to display the Health on the Net logo on their pages. In time, it is hoped that the Health on the Net logo will represent an internationally recognised stamp of quality, analogous to the BS5750 kitemark.

For details of the complete code of conduct point your browser at:

http://www.hon.ch/HONcode/Conduct.html

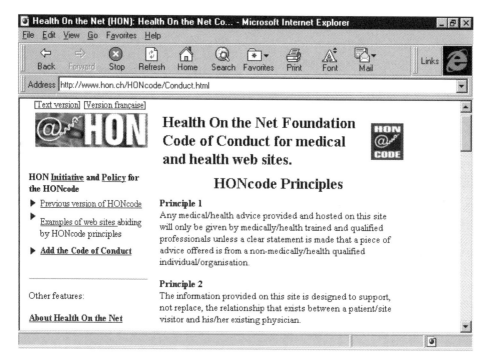

Fig. 7.7 Health on the Net Code of Conduct

To search for Web sites that comply with the code, use the Health on the Net database (Ch. 3).

Rating tools

A second way of assessing the quality of information on the Internet is to use a rating tool. A good all-purpose rating scale is the *Website Evaluation Rating Checklist*, devised by Richard Waller.[23] Using this tool, the user goes through a 60-question checklist, answering yes or no to questions such as, 'does the surfer see something meaningful within the first 8 seconds' and, if the site provides a hypertext link to another site, 'is there a description of where you are being linked to and why?' The number of 'yes' answers determines whether the site is excellent, average or problematic.

Although such a scale is fine for many sites, it is not robust and detailed enough for assessing the quality of medical information. A Web page that takes time to load may be irritating; a Web page that contains erroneous medical information may be dangerous or even life threatening!

Recognising this problem, the Health Information Technology Institute (HITI) has devised a detailed set of quality standards to help the consumer assess the quality of health information on the Internet. Credibility, content, disclosure, links, design, interactivity and caveats are the seven broad quality categories the HITI identifies. Each of these groupings is then subdivided to allow for a more accurate quality assessment to be undertaken. For example, the 'content' category has five distinct components: accuracy, hierarchy of evidence, original source stated, disclaimer, and omissions noted.

Although this work is still in progress, HITI is hoping to produce an easy-to-use tool, along the lines of a checklist, which would enable *any* Web site to be assigned a quality score. Figure 7.8 gives an idea of the type of questions the checklist will ask.

For more information, and details of the checklist, point your browser at:

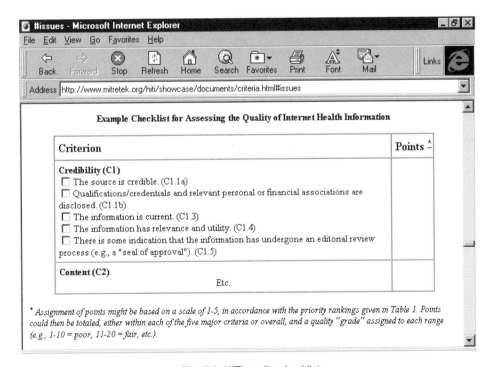

Fig. 7.8 HITI quality checklist

http://www.mitretek.org/hiti/showcase/
  documents/criteria.html

Web filtering

One other way of trying to ensure that only quality medical Web sites are delivered to your desktop is to configure your Web browser to filter out information that does not meet a defined standard.

This idea – currently being developed by a team of German physicians – is to assign labels to medical Web pages based on the PICS (Platform for Internet Content Selection) labelling scheme. Devised as a way of protecting minors from viewing inappropriate material on the Web, the PICS system enables Web authors to embed tags into a page that indicate features such as the level of nudity and violence. Subsequently, if you (or your children) try to view a page whose content exceeds the rating you have defined in your Web browser preferences, access to the page is denied.

The PICS standard, however, is flexible enough to 'label' any kind of information on the Internet. Consequently, medical Web pages could be assigned tags (med-PICS) indicating, for example, who the intended audience was, whether the information was approved or still under investigation, which country (or countries) the text is suitable for, and whether the information is deemed to be educational or promotional. Under this scheme medical professionals, associations and institutions would act as decentralised rating services and be responsible for labelling Web pages with med-PICS tags. Thus, an organisation concerned with preventive medicine and consumer protection could, for example, publish labels that identify Web pages containing dangerous or inaccurate health information.

To make use of this system the user would need to load the med-PICS rating description into his Web browser. The Microsoft Internet Explorer simply needs a text file, with the file extension .rat. Once loaded, the user is presented with a simple interface through which certain quality requirements and personal preferences can be defined. Figure 7.9 shows some of the med-PICS categories. In this example, the

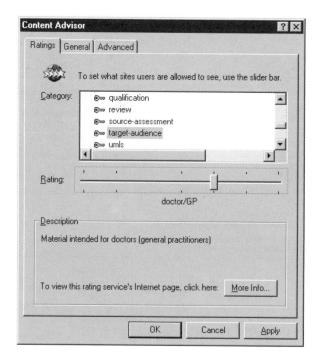

Fig. 7.9 Defining the target audience using Med-PICS

target audience has been defined as a doctor/GP. Finally, the user needs to define which labelling bureau(x) he wishes to check with before accessing any Web site.

Subsequently, when a user requests – through the browser – any Web page, the software filter not only fetches the document but *also* makes an inquiry to the label bureau(x) requesting any labels that have been assigned to that site. Depending on what the labels say, the filter may block access to that page or display a disclaimer.

Further information on med-PICS and a copy of the rating file can be obtained from:

**http://www.derma.med.uni-erlangen.de/
medpics/index.htm**

FURTHER RESOURCES

A number of Internet sites now monitor health frauds and quackery. To keep up to date with this topic, point your browser at the sites identified in Box 7.3.

CONCLUSION

As virtually anyone can set up a Web site and publish whatever they like, or post any message to discussion lists and newsgroups, *all* Internet users need to be aware of the dangers of misleading and inaccurate health information. Indeed, a study published by the Federal Trade Commission in November 1997 reported that 'in just a few hours Internet surfers identified more than 400 World Wide Web sites and numerous Usenet newsgroups that contain promotions for products and services purporting to help cure, treat or prevent heart disease, cancer, AIDS, diabetes, arthritis and multiple sclerosis'.[24] It is no coincidence that the diseases targeted are those for which there are no complete medical cures, and are thus aimed at patients who are willing to try anything. In addition to selling false hope, health fraud and quackery may also cause some

---

Box 7.3 Monitoring health frauds and quackery
Quackwatch   **http://www.quackwatch.com/**
National Council Against Health Fraud   **http://www.ncahf.org/**
Health Care Reality Check   **http://www.hcrc.org**
American Council on Science and Health   **http://www.acsh.org/**

---

patients to delay seeking proper medical diagnosis and treatment.

The crusade for quality information is further undermined when individuals and organisations post information that has an intrinsic bias to a particular pharmaceutical product, or when so-called facts are based exclusively on personal experience and anecdotes, rather than rigorous medical research and evidence.

Of course the Internet does not have a monopoly on poor and inaccurate medical information. As recently as October 1997, the *Sunday Times* ran a story with the headline 'HRT link to breast cancer proved' and stated that 'the risk of developing breast cancer [in women who take hormone replacement therapy] is 2–3 times higher, or more than double that of non-users'.[25] The research this story was based on actually concluded that the relative risk was 1.023 higher per year of use. In other words the journalist had made a one hundredfold miscalculation![26,27]

The Internet, however, is becoming *the* information source of choice for many consumers and health professionals. Consequently, if the Internet is to serve these groups effectively – by providing them with accurate and up-to-date information – the issues relating to quality must be understood, and solutions implemented. Once this happens the true value and potential of the Internet can be realised.

REFERENCES

1 Editorial 1997 The web of information inequality. Lancet 349(9068):1781–1782
2 News 1996 Internet sees growth of unverified health claims. BMJ 313(7054):381
3 Wyatt JC 1997 Commentary: Measuring quality and impact of the world wide web. BMJ 314(7098): 1879–1881 <URL: http://www.bmj.com/cgi/content/full/314/7098/1879> [Accessed 1 July 1998]
4 Impicciatore P, et al 1997 Reliability of health information for the public on the world wide web: systematic survey of advice on managing fever in children at home. BMJ 314(7098):1875–1879. <URL: http://www.bmj.com/cgi/content/full/314/7098/1875> [Accessed 1 July 1998]
5 Silberg WM, Lundberg GD, Nusacchio RA 1997 Assessing, controlling and assuring the quality of medical information on the Internet: Caveant Lector et Viewor: Let the reader and viewer beware. JAMA 277(15):1244–1245 <URL: http://www.ama-assn.org/scipubs/journals/archive/jama/vol_277/no_15/ed7016x.htm> [Accessed 4 January 1998]
6 Ojalvo HE 1996 Online advice: good medicine or cyber-quackery? American College of Physicians Online <URL: http://www.acponline.org/journals/news/dec96/cybrquak.htm> [Accessed 4 January 1998]
7 Ho KH 1996 Security and accuracy of medical information on the Internet. Canadian Medical Association Journal 154(11):1621–1622
8 News 1997 Beware the tangled Web they weave. JAMA 278(21):1724 <URL: http://www.ama-assn.org/sci-pubs/journals/archive/jama/vol_278/no_21/mn172401.htm> [Accessed 4 January 1998]
9 Nutrition Warehouse <URL: http://www.nutrition-warehouse.com/From.The.Sea.html> [Accessed 4 January 1998]
10 Triputic <URL: http://www.primenet.com/~hidden/aids.html> [Accessed 4 January 1998]
11 Federal Trade Commission. Virtual health treatments. <URL: http://www.ftc.gov/bcp/conline/edcams/miracle/index.html> [Accessed 30 November 1997]
12 Royal Rife Research Society <URL: http://www.rrrs.com/> [Accessed 30 November 1997]
13 For details of the Cancer Center Reports published by the NCC see: <URL: http://www.usc.edu/hsc/info/pr/ccr/ccr.html> [Accessed 6 January 1998]

14 Shark Cartilage Tumor Inhibitor <URL:http://home.earthlink.net/~todell/shark.htm> [Accessed 6 January 1998]
15 Miller DR et al 1997 Phase I/II trial of the safety and efficacy of shark cartilage in the treatment of advanced cancers. Proc Annu Meet Am Soc Clin Oncol 16:A173
16 Food and Drug Administration Medwatch safety summaries. <URL: http://www.fda.gov/medwatch/safety/1997/intern.htm> [Accessed 4 January 1998]
17 Food and Drug Administration – Talk paper. <URL: http://www.health.org/pressrel/feb97/3.htm> [Accessed 30 December 1997]
18 GHBinfo <URL: http://GHBinfo.com/> [Accessed 4 January 1998]
19 Some 6 months after the publication of Impicciatore's article the 'Fever as Healer' Web site was still recommending the use of alcohol as an agent for cooling a feverish child. <URL: http://www.infinite.org/aanp/articles.lay/ART.fever.tk.html> [Accessed 30 December 1997]
20 Culver JD, Gerr F, Frumkin H 1997 Medical information on the Internet: a study of an electronic bulletin board. Journal of General Internal Medicine 12(8):466–470
21 Café Herpes <URL: http://www.cafeherpe.com> [Accessed 1 July 1998]
22 Medscape <URL: http://www.medscape.com/misc/formdrugs.html> [Accessed 8 January 1998]
23 Website Evaluation Rating Checklist <URL: http://www.waller.co.uk/eval.htm> [Accessed 8 January 1998]
24 Federal Trade Commission. Health claim surf day <URL:http://www.ftc.gov/opa/9711/hlthsurf.htm> [Accessed 2 January 1998]
25 The Sunday Times 5th October 1997, p1–2
26 Collaborative Group on Hormonal Factors in Breast Cancer 1997 Breast cancer and hormone replacement therapy: collaborative reanalysis of data from 51 epidemiological studies of 52 705 women with breast cancer and 108 411 women without breast cancer. Lancet 350(9084):1047–1059
27 For a discussion of the misreporting of the research findings by the Sunday Times see: Horton R 1997 ICRF: from mayhem to meltdown. Lancet 350(9084):1043–1044

8

Consumer health information

Box 8.1 Chapter objectives

- Highlight key Web sites that provide answers to a range of typical consumer health questions.

- Discuss what impact the Internet has had on the availability of health information.

- Advance the notion that health professionals need to take on a new responsibility of directing consumers to authoritative sources of health information on the Internet.

- Discuss some of the ethical issues the Internet poses for health professionals.

INTRODUCTION

Democratising health information may, in time, come to be seen as one of the more significant changes the Internet brought about. Once the exclusive preserve of health professionals, accurate and up-to-date health information is now available to anyone who has access to the Internet. Moreover, with the development of freenets – organisations that provide free Internet access to the public – this information is available to all, irrespective of socio-economic status.

The inherent danger this situation poses is that health consumers will turn to the Internet for information rather than call their physician, and as such will be subject to inaccurate, misleading and dangerous health information, as discussed in Chapter 7. This situation will be exacerbated as more people get connected to the Internet and start using it to find health information.

One solution to this problem is for health professionals to become more Internet-aware and take on the responsibility of directing patients to those health sites which are accurate and authoritative, and able to present the information in a format which the lay person can readily understand. Moreover, taking a proactive stance on the role of the Internet gives a clear signal that information found here can, and perhaps should, be fed into the doctor/patient relationship.

The purpose of this chapter is to consider the type of information the typical patient seeks, and then highlight some of the sites that best answer these questions.

PATIENT QUESTIONS

Where can I find information about a particular illness?

Healthfinder   **http://www.healthfinder.gov/**
Health Touch   **http://www.healthtouch.com/ level1/hi_toc.htm**

A report in the *New York Times* in June 1997[1] estimated that one third of *all* searches conducted on the Internet are for health information. Although this survey does not specify which search tools are being used to find this information, research from other organisations clearly shows that Internet searchers are using the popular, non-subject specific tools such as AltaVista and Yahoo![2] When looking for health information, however, the shortcomings associated with this method of searching become all too evident:

- Too many resources are suggested. A search of AltaVista for information about meningitis points the searcher to over 9000 resources.
- Irrelevant resources are identified. A search of AltaVista for information about migraine directs you to the 'Migraine Boy' World Wide Web site. Migraine Boy is a cartoon character.
- Inaccurate and/or misleading information may also be retrieved. Among the results of a search for information about arthritis was Dr Burke's Healing Stones Web site,

where the minerals rhodonite – the 'stone of love' – and blue lace were described as effective therapies for arthritic sufferers.[3] A search of MEDLINE and the Cochrane Database of Systematic Reviews found no evidence to support these claims.

To help address these problems the US Office of Disease Prevention and Health Promotion has created the Web service Healthfinder. Healthfinder acts as a gateway to selected sources of health information that are accurate *and* suitable for consumers.

For example, on searching for information on meningitis, Healthfinder recommends just four key resources: included here is the Meningitis Foundation of America – where a detailed 'Frequently Asked Questions about Meningitis' can be found – and a fact sheet produced by the National Institute of Allergy and Infectious Diseases (NIAID) entitled 'Cryptococcal meningitis' (Figs 8.1 and 8.2).

If the resources suggested by Healthfinder do not fully answer your query, another useful source of patient information is the Health Touch WWW site. This site provides an extensive list of specialty and disease categorised patient information leaflets, derived exclusively from professional organisations. The documents are deliberately low on graphics and presented in a format appropriate for printing and distribution. Each document also states the full bibliographic source details and the date when it was last revised. A search for 'prostate cancer', for example, identified seven leaflets, including 'Symptoms and Diagnosis of Prostate Cancer', authored by the National Cancer Institute and 'Benign Prostatic Hyperplasia (BPH) and Prostate Cancer: No Apparent Relation' written by the National Kidney and Urologic Diseases Information Clearinghouse.

Where can I find out more information about a drug I have been prescribed?

US Pharmacopoeia Database

http://www.intelihealth.com/IH/

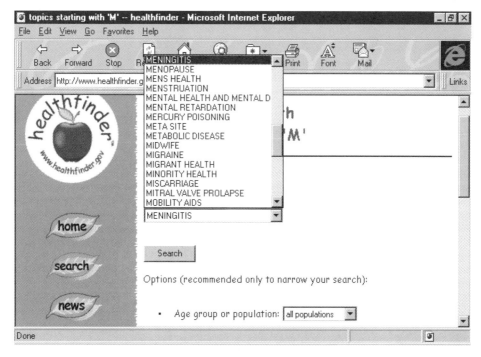

Fig. 8.1 Searching the Healthfinder database

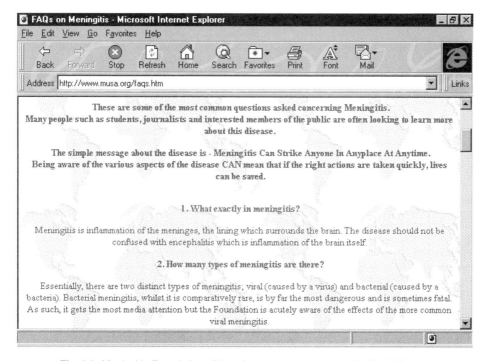

Fig. 8.2 Meningitis Foundation of America – source suggested by Healthfinder

Research shows that around 50% of all patients fail to comply with the medication regimen they are prescribed.[4] The reasons for this are numerous, but a common theme for increasing compliance is for health professionals to provide their patients with more information about the drugs they are being prescribed.[5,6] Although this is best achieved through the patient–physician consultation, if a patient requires more information, or wants some printed information for reference purposes, the US Pharmacopoeia Web site will be of use.

The US Pharmacopoeia – produced by the US Pharmacopeial Convention – provides patients with accurate and authoritative drug information in a format which is clear and jargon free. Visitors to this site have the option to either search the database (by trade or generic name) or browse through an alphabetical listing of drugs. Once a drug has been selected from the database, the information presented is in three parts: general advice for the patient (what to know about your medication and what to ask your doctor?), patient education leaflets that describe the use and side effects of this type of drug, and medicine charts that show the dosage variations, with pictures of the various pills.

For example, the migraine sufferer who has been prescribed sumatriptan is informed that the drug should be taken 'at the first sign that the headache is coming ... but if you do not feel much better in 2 to 4 hours after a tablet is taken, do *not* take any more of this medicine for the same migraine'. Instruction is also provided on how the tablets should be taken – 'do not break, crush, or chew the tablets before swallowing them' – and all known side effects are clearly listed. From a patient's perspective one of the very useful aspects of this pharmacopoeia is the way in which the adverse effects are divided into those that require 'immediate medical attention' and those where medical attention is 'not required'(Fig. 8.3).

Information in the US Pharmacopoeia is derived from a peer-review consensus process that involves medical specialty and professional practice advisory panels comprised of volunteers who objectively evaluate published data on drug products.

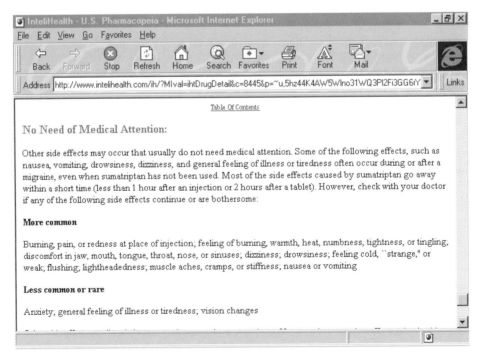

Fig. 8.3 USP Pharmacopoeia – adverse effects of sumatriptan

How long will I have to wait for my operation?

HMIS
http://www.open.gov.uk/hmis/waitime.htm
NHS Performance Tables
http://www.open.gov.uk/doh/tables96.htm

Following the publication of the Patients' Charter in the UK, much attention has been afforded to the issue of waiting times, and how these can be reduced. Leaving aside the issue of resources, one of the key components for addressing this objective is the need for the NHS to compile and publish accurate and up-to-date information on waiting times.

For patients requiring treatment in Wales this information is now available on the Internet at the HMIS Web site. Browseable by medical specialty, each list contains waiting times – down to consultant level – and shows outpatient, inpatient, day-case and combined wait. Figure 8.4 shows that a patient requiring a hip replacement will have a wait of 4 weeks if the referral is made with Mr Hunter at Llandudno General Hospital. In contrast, an appointment with Mr Wootton at Wrexham Maelor Hospital would necessitate a 41-week wait (1997 figures).

Although waiting times are not the only factor that influences which consultant a patient is referred to, making waiting time information publicly available demystifies the referral system and, in so doing, enhances the doctor/patient relationship.

Patients requiring hospital treatment in other parts of Great Britain can be referred to the NHS Performance Tables. Although not as detailed as the HMIS pages, they nevertheless give some indication of *average* wait times.

The data in these tables is arranged hierarchically by NHS Region, by NHS Trust, and finally by specialty. Looking at patients awaiting trauma and orthopaedic surgery, the NHS Tables show that in 1996 Frimley Park Hospital NHS Trust saw 49% of patients within 13 weeks of a GP referral, whilst Epsom Healthcare NHS Trust managed to see 96% of referrals within the same time (Fig. 8.5). Although these figures relate to past performance, rather than current, you can look at the

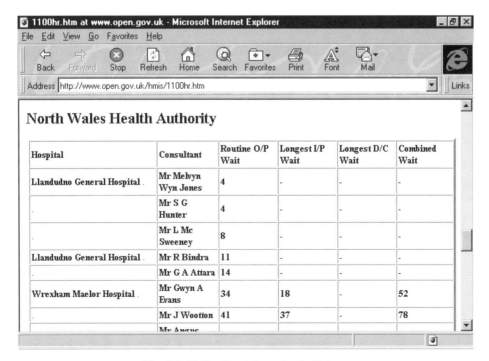

Fig. 8.4 Waiting time information in Wales

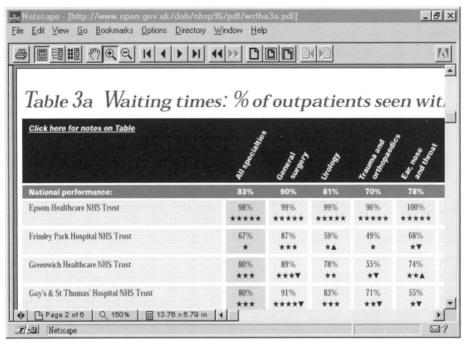

Fig. 8.5 NHS Performance Tables

previous 2 years' data on this Web site to get a clearer idea of established trends.

Is there an online doctor?

Ask the Doc   http://www.intelihealth.com/

CyberDocs   http://www.cyberdocs.com/

There are occasions when a patient may require an answer to a specific medical question but feels unable to ask his/her general practitioner or family physician. The reasons for this may be numerous: embarrassment at asking the same question twice, a wish to avoid 'wasting the doctor's time', or simply a need to get a second opinion. In recognition of these needs, the Johns Hopkins University School of Medicine in Baltimore has established the Ask the Doc interactive Web service.

The Ask the Doc service allows anyone to either mail a question to the team of 'dedicated experts', or review the answers to frequently asked questions posed by other visitors to this site. The site makes clear that not every question will be answered, and that the broader the topic the more likely you are to receive an answer.

What is reassuring about this service is that all the answers given are attributed to a named author. For example, on the day I reviewed this service there was a featured question and answer on the effectiveness of Proscar in reducing prostate gland size (Fig. 8.6). In addition to the fairly detailed reply there was a short biography of the doctor who authored the answer. In this instance I was informed that 'Jonathan P. Jarow, M.D., is Associate Professor of Urology at the Brady Urological Institute at the Johns Hopkins Medical Institution' and that 'he has a special interest in male reproductive and sexual function'. Any patient (or physician) who is still unsure of the credibility of the answer can run a search on MEDLINE to see if the cited author has published on this topic. In this case, MEDLINE identified 62 papers by Professor Jarow, most of which dealt with the male reproductive function.

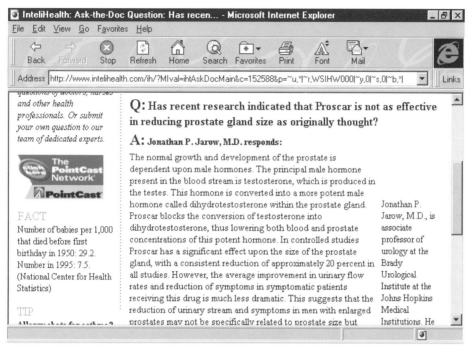

Fig. 8.6 Ask the Doc Web site – Johns Hopkins University Medical School

The Ask the Doc site publishes answers to about five questions every week. As would be expected, the nature of these varies enormously. Thus on one day the site may provide an answer to the question, *'What should I look for in choosing an over-the-counter medication for a cold?'* and on the following day deal with a far more specific query such as *'Where and how can I get the test for the colon cancer gene defect carried by Ashkenazi Jews?'* Although all the questions (and answers) can be browsed, the archive search option is a more effective way to exploit this resource.

A more interactive (and expensive) Internet medical service is provided by CyberDocs. For a fee of $50.00 Internet users can log on to this service and participate in a live one-to-one chat session with a US-registered physician (Fig. 8.7).

To use this service patients click on the Virtual Housecall button and, after submitting credit card details and providing some basic information about their medical history and details of the current health problem, are taken to the 'Doctors Office' for a consultation. If the consultation determines that medication is required, this information will be passed to a local pharmacy where it can be collected or delivered to the patient's preferred location. The entire consultation is performed via the Web browser and keyboard. No additional software is required.

CyberDocs is not meant to replace traditional physician visits. Indeed, recognising the limitations of the service – namely the inability to perform a physical examination over the Internet – CyberDocs 'mandates' users of this service to attend a follow-up session with an office-based physician, clinic or hospital emergency department. Further, this virtual doctor service is really only for minor conditions. Anyone who is experiencing chest pain, shortness of breath, abdominal pain or head or neck ache is advised to seek – in person – an immediate medical consultation, as 'Cyberdocs is not equipped to differentiate serious from non-serious forms of the above mentioned symptoms'.

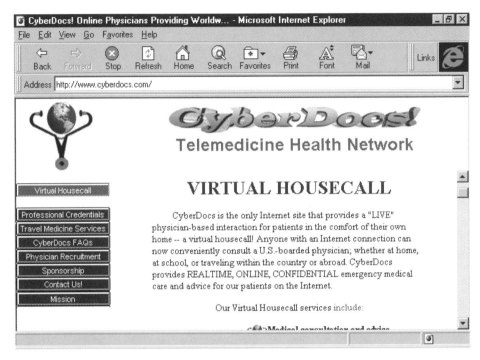

Fig. 8.7 CyberDocs

Can I identify other individuals who have a medical condition similar to my own?

MedHelp International
http://www.medhelp.org/network.htm

Contact-a-Family
http://www.cafamily.org.uk/

Numerous studies exist that demonstrate the value of encouraging patients – and their relatives – to participate in self-help groups.[7-9] One study that looked at ovarian cancer support groups concluded that, with the low rate of cure and high rate of relapse, 'psychological interventions to support patients emotionally, and to enhance their quality of life, should be considered an important complement to medical care'.[10]

Using the Internet it is possible to communicate with fellow patients through specialised discussion lists and newsgroups (Ch. 6). These forums, however, lack the intimacy that small self-help groups can provide. Indeed, figures from the Newsgroup Information Center suggest that a posting mailed to *alt.support.cancer* is read by around 10 000 people.[11]

A more personal approach to patient support has been adopted by MedHelp International. MedHelp is a non-profit organisation whose aim is to put patients in touch with other patients 'for the purpose of sharing information and support'. This objective is met through the provision of a network database which provides details – geographical location and e-mail addresses – of people who have similar medical conditions. For example, a search of this database for 'breast cancer' identifies 17 individuals, from the USA, Canada and Australia, who are willing to communicate with other women who have this condition.

To be added to the database visitors to this site complete a registration form where they disclose their e-mail address and their illness or disease. Although at the time of writing the database is fairly small – around 2000 people – and as these individuals have taken the trouble to register themselves for this service it can be inferred that the majority of requests for help and support will be answered.

As with any patient-led support service, users of MedHelp should be reminded that any information received via this network may be inaccurate and/or misleading, and consequently should be treated with caution.

For parents who are managing a child with a special need or disability, the Contact-a-Family Web site may also prove a useful resource. This site provides information on numerous medical conditions and syndromes that affect children, along with contact details of family support networks. All the information provided is written in a clear, unambiguous fashion and formatted in a way that makes it ideal for printing out and passing on to parents (Fig. 8.8). (Note: a small subscription fee is levied to access this service.) For details see:

http://www.cafamily.org.uk/form.html

Is travel health information available on the Internet?

Shoreland Travel Health Information

http://www.tripprep.com/index.html

In an age when international travel is commonplace, access to up-to-date travel health information is a frequent need. One of the best sources on the Internet for this information is provided by the Shoreland Travel Health Online Web site.

Drawing information from the Centers for Disease Control and Prevention, the World Health Organization, the US Department of State and various medical news and travel media sources, this service provides consumers with current and authoritative information on the health situation in over 500 countries.

For example, on following the hypertext link to Zambia you can identify what immunisations you need, what specific concerns have

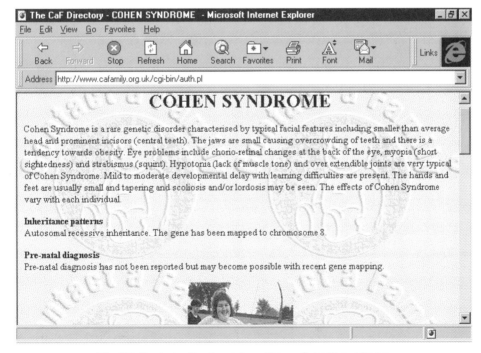

Fig. 8.8 Contact-a-Family – information on Cohen's syndrome

been identified – the climate aggravates chronic sinusitis – and what the current health situation is. On accessing this site in January 1998, I was alerted to the fact that a recent outbreak of rabies had occurred in the district of Mongu and that an outbreak of anthrax has affected at least 70 people in the Western Province. All the information cited is attributed to the appropriate source and, most importantly, is stamped with the date when the information was posted (Fig. 8.9).

Is first aid information available on the Internet?

US Dept. of Labor

http://www.medaccess.com/first_aid/ FA_TOC.htm

Evidence shows that the outcome of a patient who has suffered a heart attack is very closely related to the speed in which thrombolytic therapy can be administered. The key factor in this equation, however, is how quick-

ly the patient – or his family – can recognise the onset of a myocardial infarction. Indeed, a recent study in the *Medical Journal of Australia* found that over 50% of acute MI patients delay seeking treatment by 6 hours or more.[12] Such delay can be minimised through better patient education and developing a greater awareness of basic first aid.

One site on the Internet that discusses a whole range of medical emergencies – including cardiopulmonary resuscitation – is the First Aid Book produced by the US Department of Labor, Mine Safety and Health Administration. Taking the form of a hypertext book, this Web site is divided into 12 sections and covers everything from basic anatomy and patient assessment through to advanced CPR and the management of the haemorrhaging patient.

Written in a clear, bullet-point style, the purpose of the site is to provide a practical manual to deal with any common medical emergency. Where appropriate the text is enhanced by clear line diagrams. Figure 8.10 shows an illustration of the dressing which

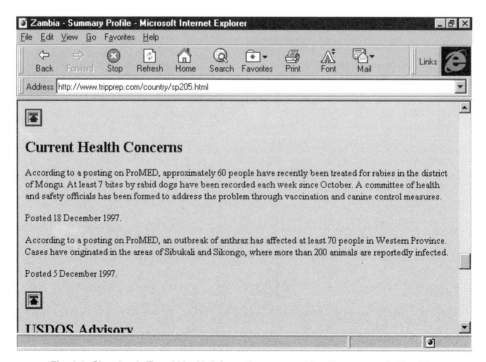

Fig. 8.9 Shorelands Travel Health Information – current health concerns in Zambia

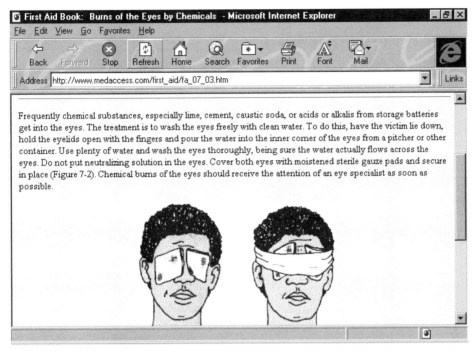

Fig. 8.10 The First Aid Book. Chemical burn to the eye – applying a dressing

should be applied to someone who has suffered a chemical burn to the eye.

THE INFORMED PATIENT: ETHICAL DILEMMAS

There is a belief that an informed patient – someone who understands things such as treatment options and long-term prognosis – is a good patient. Undoubtedly the Internet provides the opportunity for *all* patients to become more informed about their health and thus play a more active part in the health care process.

Widespread access to health information, however, will exacerbate the existing conflicts between patients' expectations of health care and what the system can afford to deliver. For example, a multiple sclerosis patient who searches the Internet MEDLINE service PubMed for information about this condition, will find an article by Rudick[13] with the following abstract:

Conclusions: The primary clinical outcome for the IFN (interferon) beta-1a clinical trial underestimated clinical benefits of treatment. Results in this report demonstrate that IFN beta-1a treatment is associated with robust, clinically important beneficial effects on disability progression in relapsing MS patients.

As this research was published in the journal *Neurology*, the official journal of the American Academy of Neurology (AAN) the data can be considered authoritative.

Interferon beta, however, does not come cheap. A paper by Walley[14] calculated that the cost of one year's treatment is around £10 000. Taking the AAN figures that this drug would help about 45% of those with the disease, the total cost of treating this percentage of UK multiple sclerosis patients would be £380m a year – about 10% of the total national drugs bill. Despite claims by successive Secretaries of State for Health that patients will always receive the drugs they need, it is difficult to believe that available resources would permit this level of expenditure. Consequently, the rationing of health care which has *always* existed will, as a consequence of the Internet, become more transparent.

It can also be anticipated that as patients become more aware of new, alternative and better treatment options, more doctors will find themselves subjected to charges of medical negligence. In law negligence is defined as 'the breach of duty to use reasonable care, as a result of which there is damage to another'.[15] To prove this it must be shown that, on the balance of all probabilities, injury to the patient resulted from the negligent act of the doctor.

In the context discussed here a doctor could be sued for negligence if the treatment given to a patient was contrary to accepted best practice. For example, a mother whose preterm baby did not survive birth could sue the medical team for negligence if, prior to the delivery, corticosteroid therapy had not been administered. Clear and *accessible* evidence, in the form of a systematic review in the Cochrane Library, states that antenatal administration of corticosteroids to women expected to deliver preterm 'reduces mortality, respiratory distress syndrome and intraventricular haemorrhage in preterm infants. No adverse consequences of this policy have been identified'.[16]

CONCLUSION

To help consumers navigate the Web effectively, health professionals will need to become 'cyber-savvy'. Directing patients to appropriate sources of information, highlighting the possible dangers of medical misinformation and quackery, and introducing the notion that all information should be critically appraised, are new responsibilities which the Internet will impose on health professionals. The Internet will also heighten the debate about health-care rationing as awareness of new (and expensive) treatments increases. It can also be assumed that a greater number of claims for medical negligence may result, some of which will be attributed to the widespread availability of health information.

On the other hand, the Internet provides health consumers with an opportunity to become informed participants in the health-care process. Using the resources discussed in this chapter health consumers can begin to tap into the wealth of information that is now available. Although the Internet can in no way replace the health professional, used effectively, I believe it can *enhance* the doctor/patient relationship.

REFERENCES

1 New York Times <URL: http://nytsyn.com/live/week/178_062797_160012_17232.html> [Accessed 3 July 1997]

2 Relevant Knowledge <URL: http://www.relevantknowledge.com/rk/press/release/10_13_97.html> [Accessed 26 October 1997] This survey showed that Yahoo! was the most popular site on the Internet, attracting some 14.5 million visitors in September 1997. Other search tools in the 'Top Web sites' includes AltaVista, Lycos and Infoseek.

3 Dr Burke's Healing Stones <URL: http://www.lotushealth.com/balls/healingstones.htm> [Accessed 21 November 1997]

4 Wright EG 1993 Non-compliance – or how many aunts has Matilda? Lancet 342(8876):909–913

5 Bebbington PE 1995 The content and context of compliance. International Clinical. Psychopharmacology 9 (suppl. 5):41–50

6 Griffith S 1990 A review of the factors associated with patient compliance and the taking of prescribed medicines. British Journal of General Practice 40:114–116

7 Montazeri A 1996 A descriptive study of a cancer support group. European Journal of Cancer Care (Engl) 5(1):32–37

8 Guidry JJ, Aday LA, Zhang D, Winn RJ 1997 The role of informal and formal social support networks for patients with cancer. Cancer Practice 5(4):241–246

9 Hemsley R 1997 The value of support. Nursing Times 93(9):28

10 Sivesind DM, Baile WF 1997 An ovarian cancer support group. Cancer Practice 5(4):247–251

11 Readership of alt.support.cancer **<URL: http://sunsite.unc.edu/usenet-i/groups-html/alt.support.cancer.html>** [Accessed 21 November 1997]

12 Dracup K, McKinley SM, Moser DK 1997 Australian patients' delay in response to heart attack symptoms. Medical Journal of Australia 166(5):233–236

13 Rudick RA et al 1997 Impact of interferon beta-1a on neurologic disability in relapsing multiple sclerosis. The Multiple Sclerosis Collaborative Research Group (MSCRG). Neurology 49(2):353–363

14 Walley T, Barton S 1995 A purchaser perspective of managing new drugs: interferon beta as a case study. BMJ 311(7008):796–799

15 British Medical Association 1992 Rights and responsibilities of doctors. BMJ Publishing p. 19

16 Crowley P 1996 Corticosteroids prior to preterm delivery. Cochrane Database of Systematic Reviews **<URL: http://www.cochrane.co.uk/abstracts/ab000065.htm>** [Accessed 18 February 1998]

9

The future

Box 9.1 Chapter objectives

- Examine some of the medical decision support tools that are emerging on the Internet.

- Explore the potential of telemedical applications being delivered over the Internet.

- Examine whether the Internet infrastructure – the wires and cables – is big enough to satisfy current and future demand for Internet services.

INTRODUCTION

The cliché that 'the only certainty is change' succinctly captures the essence of the Internet. Beginning in 1969 as a network of just four computers, the Internet has evolved into a worldwide network linking some 30 million computers and around 120 million people.[1,2]

Impressive though these figures are, they belie the fact that most of this growth has taken place within the 4 years following the release of Mosaic, the first graphical World Wide Web browser. This development not only altered the way the Internet looked, but more fundamentally it changed peoples' perceptions of *what* it could be used for. Virtually overnight the difficult, user-hostile command-line interface was replaced by one which could play audio clips, display videos and images, contain links to related documents, and launch other interactive applications. As it has become easier to use more people have sought access. In turn this has encouraged even more companies and institutions to make their resources available on the Internet.

In many ways these developments have been mirrored in the arena of medical information. Although by 1993 resources such as those at the National Institutes of Health and the National Library of Medicine could be accessed through applications such as Gopher and Telnet, the majority of sites that have been discussed in this book had no such presence on the Internet. Moreover, the idea that you could use the Internet to simulate an interactive patient encounter, or attend a virtual conference, was still considered to be the stuff of science fiction. Within the space of 2 years both of these ideas, and countless others, have been realised.

This chapter will look at new uses of the Internet in the context of health care, and indicate how these are being used to improve patient care.

MEDICAL DECISION SUPPORT SYSTEMS

In an attempt to minimise the incidence of misdiagnosis, physicians are increasingly looking to decision support systems to corroborate their findings and/or highlight anomalies and errors. In recent months some of these support systems have begun to appear on the Internet. Three of the most significant are described below.

DXplain

http://lcs-dxplain.mgh.harvard.edu/dxp/dxp
  (Password required)

http://www.lcs.mgh.harvard.edu/dxpdemo/
  start.htm (Demonstration site)

DXplain is a decision support system that uses a set of clinical findings – signs, symptoms and laboratory data – to produce a ranked list of diagnoses. DXplain also provides reasons why a particular disease might be considered, suggests what further clinical information should be collected to support the diagnosis, and lists any clinical manifestations that would be unusual or atypical for each of the specific diseases.

To use the system the physician completes a Web-based form where, after some basic demographic data about the patient has been entered, the user is able to input any clinical findings or manifestations that are deemed relevant. If a term is entered that DXplain does not recognise, alternative headings are suggested. Similarly, if a broad, generic term is entered, narrower and more specific terms are suggested. For example, although the term 'headache' is acceptable, DXplain has nine narrower and more precise terms in its database. When all the findings have been entered on the form the user clicks on the 'List Possible Diseases' button (Fig. 9.1). In this example, DXplain calculated that there was sufficient information to 'strongly support' a diagnosis of bacterial meningitis (Fig. 9.2).

At this juncture DXplain justifies how this decision was reached – fontanelle tenseness, neck stiffness and hypersomnia strongly support a diagnosis of bacterial meningitis – as well as providing further information about the disease and a list of bibliographic references for further reading.

Developed by Massachusetts General Hospital, the DXplain system contains information on over 5000 clinical manifestations, along with detailed descriptions of around 2000 diseases. Internet access to DXplain is currently in beta phase and is available without charge to medical institutions or licensed physicians.

Hepaxpert

http://www.ping.at/hepax

The Hepaxpert program makes available precise and exhaustive interpretations of hepatitis serologic results. Via a World Wide Web form, the user inputs the results of a hepatitis test and submits this for analysis (Fig. 9.3). Results are returned by e-mail within 24 hours.

As the knowledge base of Hepaxpert contains 13 'if-then' rules for hepatitis A, and 106 rules for hepatitis B serology, all possible combinations of serological test results – including

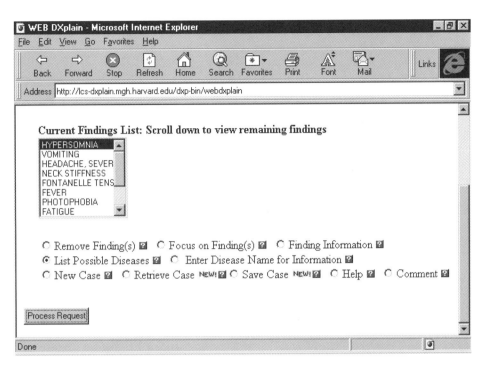

Fig. 9.1 DXplain – list of findings

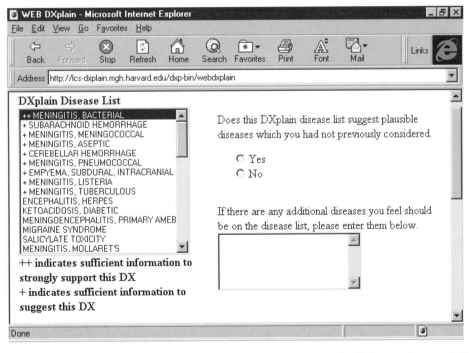

Fig. 9.2 DXplain – based on these findings, a diagnosis of bacterial meningitis is strongly supported

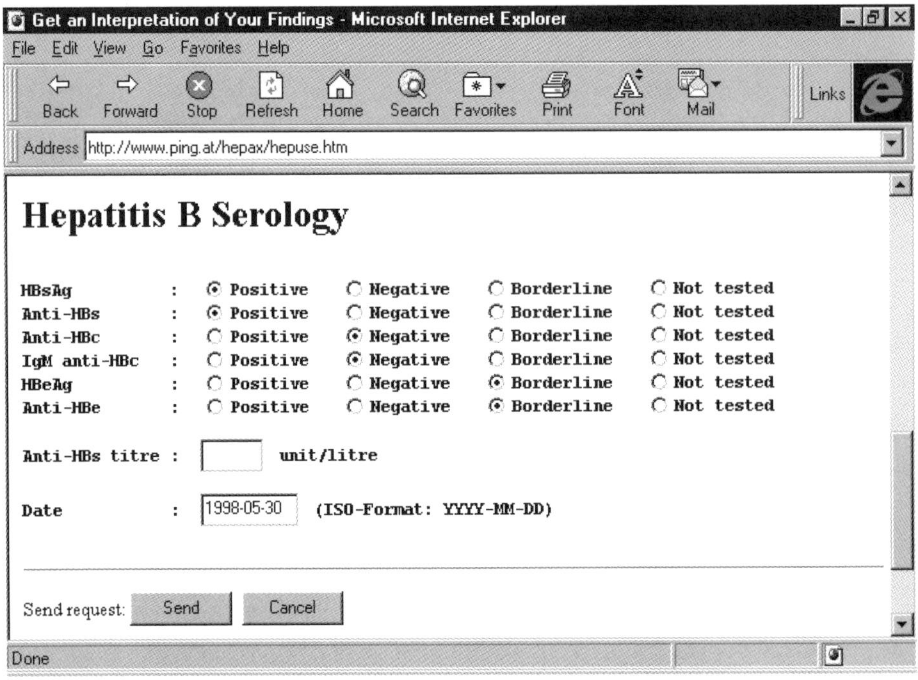

Fig. 9.3 Hepatitis B serology results submitted to Hepaxpert

rare and complex ones – can be interpreted. These rules also allow for improbable or even impossible test results to be identified.

For example, on submitting the hepatitis B serology results shown in Figure 9.3, Hepaxpert reported that:

The simultaneous occurrence of HBs-antigen and anti-HBs antibodies, with negative IgM anti-HBc antibodies, is a rare event in the natural course of a hepatitis B virus infection. This constellation of findings may be attributed to one of the following causes: (a) circulating HBsAg-anti-HBs immune complexes, (b) hepatitis B virus infection coinciding with a hepatitis B vaccination or injection of HB-hyperimmune globulin, or (c) reinfection with a hepatitis virus B with a different HBsAg subtype. Blood and secretions (saliva, sperm, breast milk) of such patients are to be regarded as infectious.

If the turnaround time for results is unacceptable, a copy of the Hepaxpert program can be purchased. The price and ordering details are available from the Web page cited above.

Computerised Medical Diagnosis

http://www.cmd.sci.fi/

Computerised Medical Diagnosis is another online diagnostic software tool that has been designed to give the possible diagnostic picture of a disease based on various symptoms, signs and physical findings.

As with DXplain, the physician uses a Web-based input form (Fig. 9.4) to indicate various signs and symptoms. For example, in the Diagnosis of Gastrointestinal Disorders program, indicating that the patient has heartburn, abdominal pain and has suffered weight loss results in the expert system suggesting a diagnosis of gastro-oesophageal reflux. Once a diagnosis has been suggested the system identifies other conditions that are associated with that disorder, as well as indicating how the diagnosis can be confirmed. In the gastro-oesophageal reflux example the program suggested that 'diagnosis should be done by endoscope, manometry, pH monitoring, and Bernstein acid perfusion'.

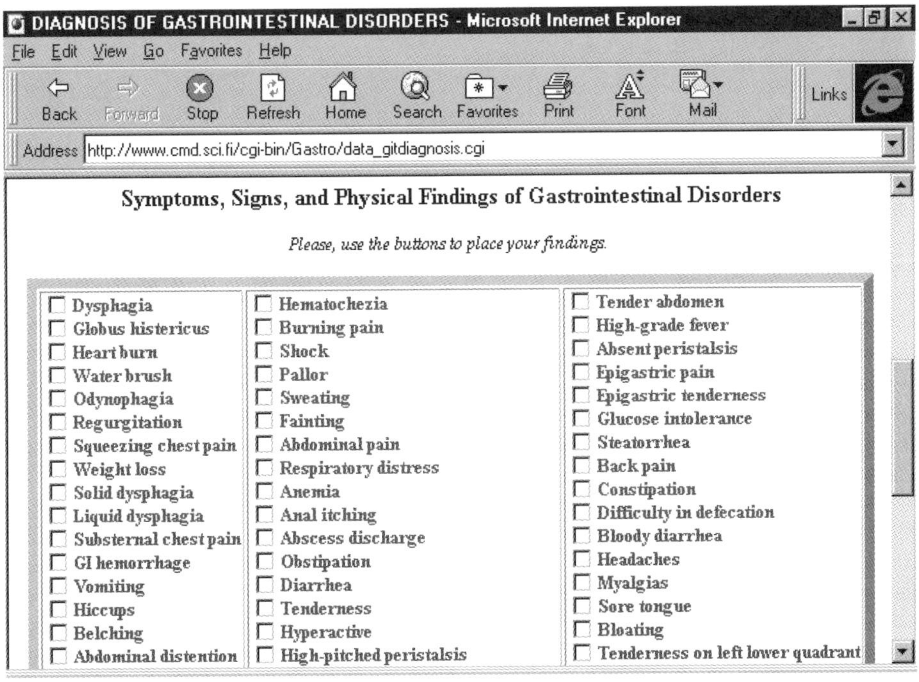

Fig. 9.4 Signs and symptoms form for the Diagnosis of Gastrointestinal Disorders program

In addition to the gastrointestinal program, CMD has also developed a software system for diagnosing pulmonary disorders and is currently writing another program to help physicians diagnose disorders of the ear, nose and throat.

Access to this site is password controlled. Weekly passwords are available for $10.00.

ONLINE MEDICAL CALCULATORS

A range of medical calculators can now be found on the Internet, all of which can help health professionals in their day-to-day work.

Obstetrics and Gynaecology Toolbox

http://www.cpmc.columbia.edu/resources/ obgyntools/

Developed by John Morrow, a Fellow of the American College of Obstetricians and Gynecologists, the 'Ob and Gyn' toolbox contains six online calculators, including a gestational age calculator, a creatinine clearance estimator and an endometriosis score calculator. This latter determines a patient's endometriosis score and stage, according to the criteria devised by the American Fertility Society. Figure 9.5 shows part of the form that needs to be completed to determine the endometriosis stage.

All the calculators that have a date function are Year-2000 compliant.

Heart Attack Survival Calculator

http://www.mei.com/resource/calculator

Based on 21 user-defined variables, the Heart Attack Survival Calculator determines a patient's survival probability following a heart attack. The definable variables include a Glasgow Coma score, respiration rate, and a range of laboratory results (Fig. 9.6). Detailed help is available for every variable.

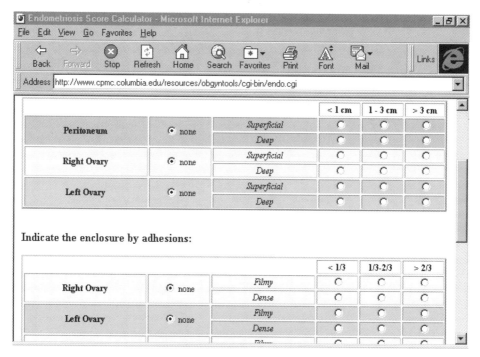

Fig. 9.5 Endometriosis score calculator – part of the 'Ob and Gyn Toolbox'

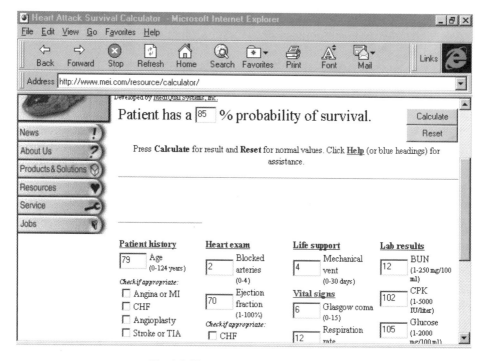

Fig. 9.6 Heart attack survival calculator

To use this calculator your Web browser must support Java applets.

Scientific Calculator

http://www.parallax.co.uk/~rolf/Calculator/

In addition to the usual calculator functions, this fully featured scientific calculator includes trigonometry functions, logarithms, factorials and 12 levels of parentheses. By mouse-clicking on the 'HEX' key the calculator loads a new keypad which can be used for performing logical calculations (Fig. 9.7).

To use this calculator your Web browser must support Java applets.

TELEMEDICINE ON THE INTERNET

Telemedicine can be defined as the use of telecommunications technologies to facilitate health-care delivery. Dating back to the 1920s, when ship-to-shore radios were used by doctors to assist with medical emergencies at sea, telemedicine has advanced to the point where remote doctor/doctor or doctor/patient consultations can now take place over the Internet.

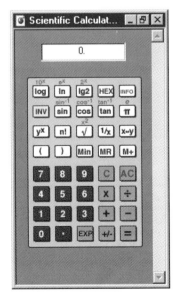

Fig. 9.7 Scientific calculator – running as a Java applet

Internet telemedicine can take various forms. In its simplest form the Internet may be used to store and forward (by e-mail or FTP) an X-ray or ECG tracing from one doctor to another. On the other hand, the Internet can be used to connect geographically remote health professionals in live video teleconsultations. EURODOC, described below, is a good example of this latter form of telemedicine.

EURODOC

http://www.artma.com/eurodoc/ Summary.html

The EURODOC initiative enables an expert to participate in a surgical procedure from any remote location. Using a technology known as 'augmented reality', an image is constructed at remote sites that merges virtual data structures (bone segments and surgical instruments) with live video data from the operating microscope. Stereotactic navigational data is also transmitted to the remote surgeons.

Because most of the graphics are compiled on the local computer, existing low-bandwidth networks (the Internet) can be used. For example, only the 3D coordinates defining rigid body movements, rather than the images themselves, are transmitted over the network.

The first surgical teleconsultation that used real-time stereotactic data was performed in August 1996, when a patient suffering from a post-traumatic deformity with multiple comminuted midface fractures was reosteotomized with the aid of remote image-guided surgery. Surgeons, separated by more than 500 kilometres, discussed the intraoperative position with regard to symmetry, hard/soft tissue relationships and occlusal details.[3]

TeleMed

http://bluemountain.acl.lanl.gov/TeleMed/ architecture.html

The purpose of the TeleMed project is to make the knowledge and experience of the pulmonary specialists at the National Jewish Medical and Research Center (NJC) in Denver,

Colorado, available to a wider audience. To achieve this, staff at non-specialist centres send chest X-rays by FTP to a national radiographic repository. Specialists from the NJC can then retrieve these images and analyse them.

What makes this telemedicine system unique is the fact that the retrieved X-rays are delivered to the Web browser as a Java applet. In this case the Java applet displays two images: a frontal X-ray and a transverse slice from part of the lung. When any part of the frontal X-ray is selected (by pointing and clicking with the mouse) the corresponding slice is displayed in the adjacent panel (Fig. 9.8).

Armed Forces Institute of Pathology (AFIP)

http://www.afip.org/telepathology/
index.html

Telepathology enables a pathologist practising in a geographical distant site to consult another pathologist for a second opinion, or other pathologists who are experts on particular disease processes. AFIP, with 125 pathologists working in 22 different subspecialties, is a world leader in the practice of pathology: with telepathology this expertise can now be enjoyed throughout the world. Using the basic Internet facilities, e-mail and FTP, pathologists can forward pathology images to AFIP for diagnosis.

To make use of this facility pathologists need access to a microscope with a high-resolution camera, an image capture board and some software to manage the images. Once the image has been received, AFIP aims to report the final diagnosis to the referring pathologist within 24 hours.

No charge is made for consultations from US military establishments or for overseas contributors enrolled in military, WHO or other AFIP cooperative programs. Civilian pathologists are charged $50.00 per consultation. For further details contact AFIP at: **telepath@email.afip.osd.mil**

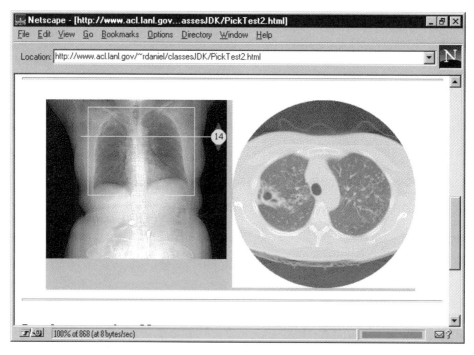

Fig. 9.8 TeleMed Java applet: when any part of the frontal X-ray is selected the corresponding slice is displayed in the adjacent panel

Further information

Highly trained specialists are an expensive and scarce resource. Telemedical applications, such as the ones described here, help ensure that they are used effectively. For more information about telemedicine, and telemedical applications on the Internet, point your Web browser at the Telemedicine Information Exchange: **http://tie.telemed.org/**

THE INFORMATION SUPERHIGHWAY

The increasing reliance upon the Internet for mail, information, education and decision support raises the issue of whether the network infrastructure is sufficiently developed to handle this volume of traffic. To assess this, we can examine current developments in both public and institutional computer networks.

Public networks

Unless you are part of an institution that has a dedicated 'feed' to the Internet (discussed below) the only way you can access it is by setting up an account with a commercial Internet provider. Once this has been established you can access their Internet 'feed' via the telephone network (Ch. 2).

Although this mode of access *is* perfectly acceptable – indeed, most of the research for this book was undertaken using a dial-up connection – as the Internet moves increasingly away from text-based sources to high-bandwidth multimedia applications, the relative slowness of the telephone connection will be exacerbated. Thus, whereas most commercial Internet providers are connected to the Internet at high speeds – Demon Internet, for example, has a 45 Mbps (megabits per second) line to the US – their customers (you and I) are connected by a modem running at either 28.8 Kbps or 56 Kbps (kilobits per second). Like any system, the Internet is only as good as its weakest link; at the moment this is the telephone line.

The obvious solution to this problem is the creation of a national high-speed computer network. In the United States such a plan is being enabled through the Next Generation Internet (NGI) initiative.

Next Generation Internet (NGI)

Figures from the US government indicate that by the year 2000 more than half of the US population is expected to have access to the Internet. To ensure that this mass of people can access the Internet and the new high-bandwidth applications that are coming online, the Next Generation Internet (NGI) initiative has been developed.

The NGI initiative is a multiagency federal research and development program which aims to develop networking technologies that can deliver data at speeds 100–1000 times faster, end-to-end, than today's Internet. Once developed, this network could support applications such as real-time telemedicine, or radiology consultation workstations which would provide remote consultation opportunities for radiation oncologists and radiologists through the use of interactive image analysis.

Speaking in his 1998 State of the Union Address, President Clinton described the Internet as 'getting kind of clogged'.[4] The NGI initiative should help mitigate this problem, and in so doing enable all Americans to 'live better and work smarter'.[5] For more information about the NGI initiative see: **http://www.ngi.gov/**

In the UK, the government has no plans to build a national high-speed computer network. Consequently, users who want faster access to the Internet must look elsewhere.

Broadband technology

Although ISDN (Ch. 2) provides reasonable access speeds to the Internet it is not broadband technology. It has been calculated, for example, that it would take 24 hours to download a 60-minute video film using ISDN lines.[6]

The solution to slow access speeds seems to lie with the cable companies, who in recent months have developed and tested the first high-speed cable modems. Although cable networks have been delivering full motion video and digital audio to television sets for a number of years, sending data back down the line has always been more problematic. Indeed, many cable companies request their customers to order pay-per-view movies and sports programming over the telephone, rather than with a cable box.

However, subscribers who live in the areas where cable Internet services are available can enjoy access speeds of up to 100 times faster than that offered by a modem. A recent article in *ZD Net* spoke of being able to download Netscape Navigator – all 25 MB of it – in just 41 seconds.[7]

One of the leading exponents of this technology is the High Velocity @Home Service. @Home provides subscribers with a cable modem, network card (10 base-T Ethernet) and a cable to connect to your data cable line. Although the monthly subscription prices are more expensive than a traditional dial-up service – typically between $35 and $55 – there are *no* telephone charges to add to this equation. With cable modems you are permanently connected to the Internet, in just the same way as a television set is always connected and ready to receive pictures.

@Home is available in selected areas of the United States, Canada, the Netherlands, Belgium and the United Kingdom. For more details – and to see if this service is available in your area – point your browser at: **http://www.home.net/**

Institutional networks

NHSnet

For health professionals working in the UK the most significant networking development is the creation of the internal NHS-wide network, NHSnet. Although its main purpose is administrative – to facilitate the growing need for organisations within the NHS family to share information – the network will also provide a high-speed access point to the Internet (NHSweb).

In addition to providing a link to the Internet, NHSweb also hosts services that are of general use to the NHS. Products currently available include the NHSweb Directory – a searchable database containing links to sites on both NHSweb and the Internet – and NHSp, which provides information on NHS personnel issues. As much of the data on NHSnet is of a highly sensitive and confidential nature the network will not actually form part of the Internet. Internet access will be via a secure one-way gateway, which will prevent ingress on to NHSnet from Internet users.

If you have an NHSnet connection further details of the services available can be found at: **http://nww.inform.nhsweb.nhs.uk**. This address will *not* work if you are not part of NHSnet.

For more general information, available to all Internet users, see:

http://www.info-com.com/nhstb/centre/

SuperJANET III

For academics in the United Kingdom the problem of access speed is being addressed with the development of SuperJANET III, an advanced high-speed optical computer network which will provide connections running at 155 Mbps.

One example of how this high-speed network is being used in the field of medical education is the Interactive Teaching Project in Surgery, developed by University College, London.[8] Via this initiative, medical students at six SuperJANET sites can watch live transmissions of surgical operations and interact with the surgical team as if they were actually in the operating theatre. Thus, this project allows a large number of students to see a wide range of operative procedures and hear and see at first hand the opinions and skills of some of the best surgeons in the UK.

Internet2

Internet2 is a collaborative effort by over 120 US universities to 'develop advanced Internet technology and applications vital to the research and education missions of higher education'.[9] Central to this is the need to create a high-performance network for the *exclusive* use of the research community. Members of the Internet2 collaboration believe that the congestion on the Internet 'has had a significant negative impact on the university research community'.[10]

Internet2 aims to develop new technologies – such as multicasting – which will be of benefit to the research community. It will not, however, replace the Internet. Internet2 will offer no access to the World Wide Web, or e-mail. Members of the Internet2 consortium will still use the Internet for these services.

Once stable Internet2 connections have been developed there are plans to transfer this technology to the commercial sector, where the benefits can be enjoyed by all. Just as the World Wide Web is a legacy of earlier investments in academic and research networks, so the legacy of Internet2 will be technology that can be adopted by the commercial sector.

For further information about Internet2 see:

http://www.internet2.edu/

CONCLUSION

The future of the Internet is one where change and evolution are its constant bedfellows. The introduction of WebTV, for example, looks likely to be the next big application to take hold on the Internet, whilst in more general terms users can expect services to become increasingly commercialised.

For health professionals, the Internet of the future will offer enhanced access to a wealth of information resources and teaching tools, and through telemedical applications and decision support systems, provide the opportunity to deliver patient care more effectively.

The size and volatility of the Internet ensures that any book on this subject can only provide a snapshot of what is available. To explore further, and truly reap the benefits the Internet can deliver, I urge all health professionals to get connected and then to spend some time exploring 'cyberspace'. The sites discussed in this book provide a good launch-pad to some of the premier health sites on the Internet. For convenience, many of the Web sites discussed in this text can be accessed from the Harcourt Brace World Wide Web site at:

http://www.hbuk.co.uk/kiley/

From this page you can also mail me with comments and questions, and suggest other interesting Internet sites that could be included in future editions.

I look forward to hearing from you.

REFERENCES

1 Net Wizards <**URL: http://www.nw.com/zone/WWW/report.html**> [Accessed 12 June 1998]
2 NUA Internet Surveys <**URL: http://www.nua.ie/surveys/how_many_online/index.html**> [Accessed 12 June 1998]
3 Millesi W 1997 Remote stereotactic visualization for image-guided surgery: technical innovation. Journal of Cranio-Maxillo-Facial Surgery 25(3):136–138
4 Clinton W State of the Union speech, 1998 <**URL: http://www.whitehouse.gov/WH/SOTU98/address.html**> [Accessed 15 June 1998]
5 Next Generation Internet <**URL: http://www.ngi.gov/overview/fast_facts.html**> [Accessed 15 June 1998]

6 Winder D Step up to the superhighway. Sunday Times 7 January 1996
7 ZD net magazine <**URL: http://www.zdnet.com/products/content/articles/199804/cable.wired/2.html**> [Accessed 15 June 1998]
8 Interactive Teaching Project in Surgery <**URL: http://av.avc.ucl.ac.uk/tltp/**> [Accessed 15 June 1998]
9 Internet2 <**URL: http://www.internet2.edu/html/faqs.html#**> [Accessed 15 June 1998]
10 Internet2 <**URL: http://www.internet2.edu/html/about_i2.html**> [Accessed 15 June 1998]

Appendix A

Finding more information

If, after reading this book, you would like to learn more about the Internet, the sources cited below are recommended starting points. For ease of use I have split these resources into two sections: first, those that can be accessed via the Internet: secondly, for readers who have not yet got connected, I have compiled a brief, annotated bibliography.

INTERNET RESOURCES

Tutorials

The first two resources cited here are both Internet-based courses which aim to help new users make effective use of the Internet. Both are free of charge and may be undertaken at your own pace.

The Online Netskills Interactive Course (TONIC)

http://www.netskills.ac.uk/TONIC

TONIC is a Web-based interactive tutorial designed to offer practical guidance on how to use the Internet. The main modules of the course are:

- exploring the Internet;
- basic networking tools, such as Telnet and FTP;
- searching the Internet;
- communicating via the Internet.

Which of these you pursue, or in what order, is entirely up to you. Once you have registered your interest to follow this tutorial you are assigned a log-in name. When you next log on, the program will 'remember' which parts of the tutorial you have already completed. As you progress through the modules you are able to test your knowledge and receive corresponding feedback.

This course has been produced by Netskills, with central funding from the Higher Education Funding Councils of England, Scotland and Wales and the Department of Education for Northern Ireland. Although it was developed for the benefit of the UK higher education community, it may be used freely for non-commercial academic purposes.

Beginners Central

http://www.northernwebs.com/bc/

Beginners Central is another Internet training workshop designed to help new Internet users 'bring order to the chaos'. Topics covered include how to search the Internet, downloading programs and contributing to discussion lists and newsgroups.

Discussion lists

The Internet Tourbus

For suggestions on interesting Internet sites to visit, subscribe to the *Internet Tourbus* discussion list. Recommended sites come with an in-depth description and analysis. In an average month the owners of the list will mail you with about five suggestions.

To subscribe, send the following e-mail:

To: listserv@listserv.aol.com
Subject   leave blank
Message subscribe TOURBUS *yourfirstname yoursurname* end

Alternatively, visit the Tourbus home page and browse through the previous tours:

http://www.tourbus.com/

NewbieNewz

**http://www.newbie.net/NewbieNewz/
subscribe.html**

This discussion list exists to serve the needs of new Internet users. Regular mailings aim to

answer most questions new users are likely to ask. On those occasions when *specific* help is required, subscribers can mail the help desk for assistance.

To subscribe to this mailing list send the following e-mail:

To: Owner-NewbieNewz@newbie.net
Subject   Leave blank
Message subscribe newbienewz end

NON-INTERNET RESOURCES

Books

The number of books that discuss the Internet is staggering. A search of the Internet Bookshop, for example (**http://www.bookshop.co.uk**), identifies more than 2000 books on this topic. I am, however, going to recommend just two:

- Schofield S The UK Internet book revised for '95. Addison-Wesley 1995 ISBN 0201877317
- Quercia V Internet in a nutshell. O'Reilly and Associates 1997 ISBN 1565923235

The first is aimed at the dial-up UK Internet market and provides an excellent introduction to the Internet. The second is advertised as 'a second-generation Internet book for readers who have already taken a spin around the Net and now want to learn the shortcuts'. In this sense it is a more advanced book that provides some useful information, particularly on features such as authoring a Web page, and setting up helper applications and plug-ins.

Journals

To keep abreast of Internet developments I would recommend subscribing to at least one Internet journal. The titles cited here are the ones I find most useful. The *Internet Magazine* and *Boardwatch* (aimed at the UK and US markets, respectively) are general-interest Internet magazines, whilst *He@lth Information on the Internet* (edited by this author) aims to provide information about how the Internet can be of practical use to health professionals.

The Internet Magazine

Priory Court, 30-32 Farringdon Lane, London EC1R 3AU

Tel: +44 (0) 181 956 3105; Fax: +44 (0) 181 956 3023

http://www.internet-magazine.com/

e-mail: internet.subs@computing.emap.co.uk
ISSN:1355-7602

Boardwatch

13949 W Colfax Ave Suite 250, Golden, CO 80401, USA

Tel: 303-235-9510; Fax: 303-235-9502

http://www.boardwatch.com

ISSN:1054-2760 -

Hea@lth Information on the Internet

Royal Society of Medicine Press, 1 Wimpole Street, London W1M 8AE

Tel: +44 (0) 171 290 2928; Fax: +44 (0) 171 290 2929

http://www.wellcome.ac.uk/healthinfo

e-mail: arvinder.ali@roysocmed.ac.uk
ISSN:1460-4140

Articles

A search of the MEDLINE database for the term 'Internet' indicates that between January 1995 and July 1998 this one database indexed more than 1100 articles on this subject. Key citations from this search are detailed below:

Ellenberger B 1995 Navigating physician resources on the Internet. Canadian Medical Association Journal 152(8):1303–1307

Glowniak JV 1995 Medical resources on the Internet. Annals of Internal Medicine 13:123–131

Jadad AR, Gagliardi A 1998 Rating health information on the Internet – navigating to knowledge or to Babel? JAMA 279(8):611–614

Pallen M 1995 Guide to the Internet. A series of four articles:
  (i)   Introducing the Internet. BMJ 311(7017):1422–1424
  (ii) Electronic mail. BMJ 311(7018):1487–1490
  (iii) The World Wide Web. BMJ 311(7019):1552–1556
  (iv) Logging in, fetching files, reading news. BMJ 311(7020):1626–1630

Silberg WM, Lundberg GD, Nusacchio RA 1997 Assessing, controlling and assuring the quality of medical information on the Internet: *Caveant Lector et Viewor:* Let the reader and viewer beware. JAMA 277(15):1244–1245

Wyatt JC 1997 Measuring the quality and impact of the world wide web. BMJ 314(7098):1879–1881

Netscape Navigator and Internet Explorer: frequently asked questions

This appendix will pose and answer the most frequently asked questions about installing, configuring and using the Web browsers Netscape Navigator and the Microsoft Internet Explorer. All commands are correct for releases 3.0 and above, running under Windows 3.x or Windows95.

Note: In this Appendix commands appear in the form **menu name | command name**. Thus **File | Save** means 'open the file menu and then select the save option'.

Where can I get the latest software releases from?

To take advantage of the latest Web features, an up-to-date Web client is essential. For example, Java Applets (computer programs which can be included on a Web page in much the same way as a graphic) can only be displayed if you are running version 2.0 (or later) of Netscape or Internet Explorer, whilst to use Microsoft's Net Meeting software – for Internet video conferencing – version 4.0 of the Internet Explorer is recommended.

The latest version of Netscape can be obtained from:

http://home.netscape.com/

The latest version of Internet Explorer can be downloaded from:

http://www.microsoft.com/ie

At these sites follow the links to the latest release appropriate to your operating system (Windows 3.1, Mac, NT etc). If a local mirror site is suggested use this for faster access.

How long does it take to FTP a copy of this software?

To a large extent this depends on which version you download, how fast your Internet connection is, and how congested (or otherwise) the network is. However, as a guide the following figures are provided:

Browser	Version	Operating system	Size	Time
Netscape	4.05	Windows95	8.5 MB	1 hour
Internet Explorer	4.0	Windows95	12.3 MB	1.5 hours

How do I install the Web browser?

Both browsers are downloaded as a self-executable archive. The Netscape file, for example, is n32e405.exe. Use the **Run** command to extract various files, including a 'setup' and a 'readme' file. After reading the 'readme' file, double-click on the setup file.

My Web browser automatically loads the Netscape/Microsoft Home Page when I connect to the Internet. How I can stop this?

As shipped, Netscape is configured to load the Netscape Home Page. To stop this select: **Options | General Preferences | Appearance | Start with blank page**.

To make the *Medical Information on the Internet* Web site your default home page select **Options | General Preferences | Appearance | Home Page Location** and enter:

http://www.hbuk.co.uk/kiley/

Users of the Internet Explorer can change their default home page by selecting: **View | Options | Navigation | Customise** and entering the URL of their choice.

How do I link to other pages, and go back to a page I have already seen?

All highlighted words (coloured or underlined) are hypertext links. Clicking on any link will load up that related page, wherever it happens to be located on the Internet. Click on the arrow buttons ← → to go back (or forward) to a page you have previously seen. If your toolbar is not visible select **Go | Forward** or **Go | Back**.

What are bookmarks?

Bookmarks are a way of recording the location of a particular Internet site. When you wish to revisit a bookmarked site you can do so without having to remember the specific URL. The Internet Explorer uses the term favourites.

How do I make a bookmark/favourite?

To bookmark any page select **Bookmarks | Add Bookmark.** To arrange the Bookmarks hierarchically select **Bookmarks | Go to Bookmark | Insert Folder.** You can then cut and paste specific bookmark entries to specific folders. For example, you may have a 'Health' folder to keep health-related sites together and a 'Search Engine' folder to facilitate easy access to your favourite search tools.

Using Internet Explorer select **Favourites | Add to Favourites**. To arrange the favourite sites in subject-related folders, use **Favourites | Organise Favourites.**

How can I save a file?

To minimise online time it makes sense to save files to disk and read them offline. In both browsers click on **File | Save As** and assign a file name and location (or accept the defaults). To read this file when you have severed your connection to your Internet provider, select **File | Open File**, and select the appropriate file.

Using Netscape it is possible to save a file to disk *without* viewing it first. To achieve this, click on a hypertext link with the **Shift** key held down.

How can I save an image?

When you save a file images are replaced by icons. However, specific images can be saved by placing your mouse pointer over the image and clicking the right-hand mouse button. From the pop-up menu select '**Save this image as**' (Netscape) '**Save Picture as**' (Internet Explorer) and enter a file name or accept the default.

How do I FTP a file through my Web browser?

FTP'ing is the same process as saving a file (**File | Save As**). If you try to view an executable file (such as a program file) the browser will realise that the file cannot be displayed, and prompt you with a <u>dialogue box</u> to supply a file name and location.

How can I print a Web page?

If the browser tool bar is visible, press the printer icon; otherwise select **File | Print**. As printing can be a relatively slow process (and therefore relatively costly), I would recommend saving the file to disk and printing it later.

When I try to connect to a <u>Telnet</u> site I get the message 'unable to find application'. What does this mean?

To run a Telnet session you must have a Telnet client, and configure the browser to load this application.

Using Netscape select **Options | General Preferences | Apps | Supporting Applications | Telnet.** Give the file name and disk location of the Telnet client.

Using Internet Explorer select **View | Options | Programs | Viewers | File type | New Type** and enter the file name and disk location of the Telnet client.

When I try to view a <u>pdf</u> file through the Web browser I get an 'application unknown' error message. What does this mean and how do I correct this?

Netscape and Internet Explorer can only display pdf files if you have a pdf client – typically the

Adobe Acrobat – installed on your computer. If this is the case you can configure your browser to launch this application automatically. (It saves you the bother of having to save the file, and then load up another piece of software.)

Using Netscape, select **Options | General Preferences | Helpers | Create New Type.** Define the **MIME type** as application and the **MIME sub-type** as pdf. Define the **File Extension** as pdf. Check the option to **Launch the Application** and define the path and file name of your <u>pdf</u> viewer, e.g. c:\acrobat3\reader\acrord32.exe.

Using Internet Explorer, select **View | Options | Programs | Viewers | File type | New Type.** Define the **Description of Type** as Adobe Acrobat, the **Associated Extension** as pdf, and the **Content type/MIME** as application/pdf. Click on the **New Actions** and **Define** and enter the path and file name of your pdf viewer.

Whenever your browser subsequently encounters a pdf file it will automatically launch the viewer. Chapter 3 has details on how to find software clients.

If I know the <u>URL</u> of a Web site can I jump straight to it?

Yes. Select **File | Open** and in the dialogue box type in the URL. As most servers on the Internet are <u>UNIX</u> based the case of the address is crucial. If an address is cited in lower case and you enter it in capitals you will receive an error message to the effect that the address cited does not exist.

Note: As both Netscape and the Internet Explorer default to the <u>HTTP</u> protocol (hypertext transfer protocol) the **http://** part of a Web address can be omitted. Thus **File | Open www.mailbase.ac.uk/** is the same as
File | Open http://www.mailbase.ac.uk/

How can I speed up the loading of Web pages?

Disabling the image capabilities dramatically reduces the time it takes to load a Web page.

Using Netscape this can be implemented by selecting **Options** and deselecting the **Auto**

Load Images option. (This is a toggle switch; if the option is marked with a ✓ images will be displayed.) On those occasions when you want to see a specific image, simply click on the image's icon.

Using Internet Explorer, Web graphics can be disabled by selecting **View | Options | General** and unchecking the **Show Pictures** option.

Some Internet providers set up a temporary cache to store Web pages and files that have recently been accessed. If the Web site you seek is already present in this cache then delivery to your desktop will be far quicker than if you have to fetch the page from the host server.

Using Netscape this facility can be implemented by selecting **Options | Network Preferences | Proxies | Manual Proxy Configuration | View** and in the HTTP proxy box enter the address of this server and its appropriate port. (This information will be supplied by your Internet provider.)

Using Internet Explorer this facility can be implemented by selecting **View | Options | Connections | Proxy server | Settings** and entering the address of the proxy server and its port number.

Despite doing the above a particular Web page still seems to be taking a long time to come through. Can I stop the transfer?

Yes. Click the red **Stop** button, if your browser toolbar is visible, or simply hit the **Escape** key on your keyboard.

Some of the graphics appear to be corrupted. Can I correct this?

Yes, by reloading the document: **View | Reload** (Netscape), **View | Refresh** (Internet Explorer).

How can I configure my browser to send and receive e-mail?

To be able to send and receive mail through your browser your Internet provider must provide **both** an SMTP (simple mail transfer protocol) server for outgoing mail and a POP3 (Post Office protocol, version 3) for incoming mail. If this is the case, then under Netscape select **Options | Mail and News Preferences** and enter the address of the SMTP server, the POP3 server, and your POP3 user name in the

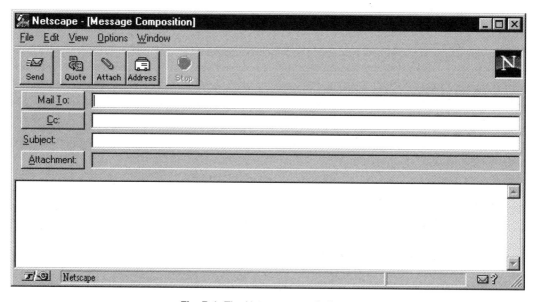

Fig. B.1 The Netscape e-mail client

appropriate boxes. Save these options. To load the Netscape Mail client select **Window | Netscape Mail**. To retrieve mail from your provider's POP3 server select **File | Get New Mail.** To send messages select **File | Send Mail in Outbox**. (Mail is composed offline.)

If your provider only offers an SMTP server for both incoming and outgoing mail Netscape can only be used to *send* mail. This is done through the **File | New Mail Message** option (Fig. B.1).

To configure Internet Explorer for e-mail select **View | Options | Programs** and select **Internet Mail** as the mail service you wish to use whilst browsing the Internet. Launch the Internet Mail client (**Go | Read Mail**), select **Mail | Options** and using the **Server** tab define the outgoing and incoming mail servers (Fig. B.2). To retrieve mail from your provider's POP3 server select **Go | Read Mail.**

How can I read usenet newsgroups through my browser?

To be able to subscribe to and read usenet newsgroups your Internet provider must provide access to an NNTP server (network news transport protocol). If this condition is met, Netscape users should select **Options | Mail and News Preferences** and enter the address of the NNTP server. The first time you connect to the NNTP server, Netscape will download a list of all available newsgroups. To load the Netscape News browser select **Window | Netscape News**. To see which newsgroups are available for subscription select **Options | Show all Newsgroups**.

To configure Internet Explorer for newsgroups select **View | Options | Programs** and select **Internet News** as the news service you wish to use whilst browsing the Internet. Launch the news client (**Go | Read News**), select **News | Options** and, using the **Server** tab, enter the address of the NNTP server. The first time you connect to this server Internet Explorer will download a list of all available newsgroups. This list can be viewed by **News | Newsgroups**. Any newsgroup you wish to subscribe to can be defined at this point.

Can I search a Web page for a particular word or phrase?

Yes. In both Netscape and Internet Explorer use the **Edit | Find** option and enter the word or phrase you wish to search for.

I want to purchase a product via the Internet. Is it safe to transmit my credit card details via my Web browser?

Yes, provided the site you are accessing uses public key cryptographic technology. This can be determined in two ways. First, Web sites that use this technology cause the browser to display a graphical key. In Netscape this can be seen by the two halves of a key – visible on every Web page – joining together (Figs B.3 and B.4). Users of Internet Explorer will see a key and padlock to indicate that you have a secure connection to that Web site (Fig. B.5).

Secondly, by selecting **View | Document Info** in Netscape and **File | Properties | Security** in Internet Explorer, details relating to the security of the site can be viewed (Fig. B.6).

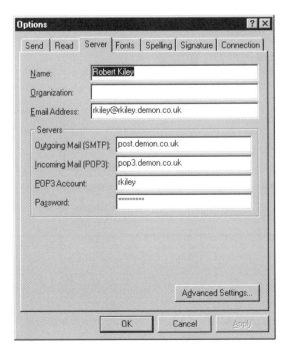

Fig. B.2 Defining your mail servers for Internet Explorer

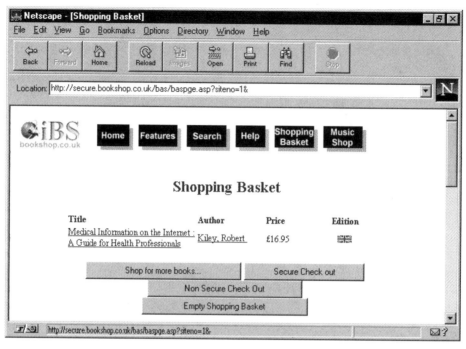

Fig. B.3 Whilst searching the IBS site, a standard insecure site is acceptable. Note the key in the bottom left-hand corner is broken

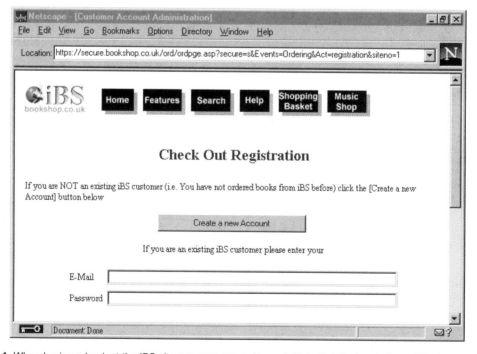

Fig. B.4 When buying a book at the IBS site a secure server is used. Note that the two halves of the key are joined

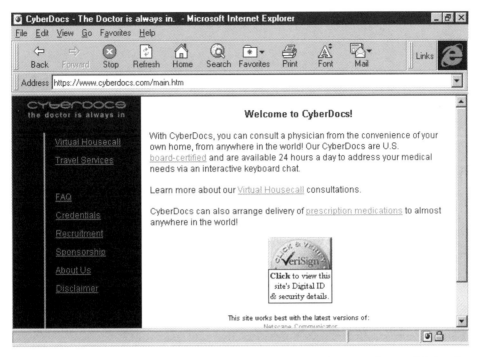

Fig. B.5 A secure site as identified by the Internet Explorer. Note the padlock at the bottom right-hand corner

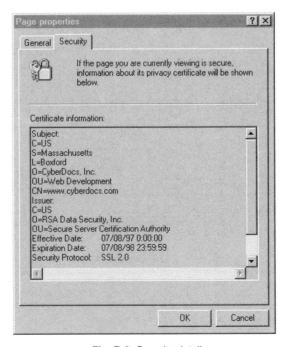

Fig. B.6 Security details

Appendix C

Optimising your computer

This appendix describes a couple of 'tweaks' you can undertake to optimise your computer's performance for Internet-specific tasks.

UPGRADING THE PROCESSOR SERIAL PORT

The serial port is where you connect the <u>modem</u> to the computer. Generally speaking, to drive modems at speeds greater than 14 400 bps (bits per second) it is recommended that your serial port is fitted with a 16550A chip. How you check this depends on what sort of computer you have.

IBM-compatibles

For IBM-compatibles you need to access the operating system (DOS) that sits below Windows. To do this, follow these instructions:

1. Exit to DOS by closing Windows.
2. At the C: prompt type 'msd'. This will run the 'Microsoft Diagnostic Program'. If this file is not in your root directory, reload Windows and use the search option within the File Manager to identify the location of the file msd.exe.
3. From the main diagnostic utility menu, select the option to examine the COM Ports.
4. At the bottom of the display you will find notification of the type of UART chip each port uses. If an 8250 chip is reported I would recommend upgrading. The cost of

replacing this chip – around £25.00 – will be recovered through faster, and therefore cheaper, Internet sessions.

Other computers

For details of how to check the port settings on other operating systems, either consult your manual or, once you have connected to the Internet, visit one of the following sites for further information:

Amiga:

http://www.omnipresence.com/Amiga/ mainpage.html

Apple:

http://www.apple.com/support

Atari:

http://www.atarimagazines.com/

REVERSING DISK COMPRESSION UTILITIES

If at some point you have compressed your hard disk (using a product such as DoubleSpace) it may be a good idea to reverse this. As files from the Internet are cached to your hard disk a compressed disk will perform this task more slowly, resulting in longer online times and higher telephone bills.

Before doing this, however, back up all your files and check that your hard disk will be big enough to accommodate the uncompressed files. If space is a problem consider 'zipping up' any program files you do not use that often, but do not wish to delete. Chapter 2, 'Installing FTP'd software', has details of various archiving (zipping) utilities.

Appendix D

Configuring TCP/IP

GENERAL INFORMATION

Table D.1 details the data required for a typical TCP/IP configuration.

FOR WINDOWS95

Although Windows95 comes with the necessary components to connect to the Internet (TCP/IP, SLIP/PPP) it is still necessary to configure them. This section details the way I set up my connection.

Note: In this Appendix commands appear in the form **menu name I command name**. Thus **Settings I Control Panel** means 'click on the settings menu and then select the control panel option'.

Step 1 Check to see if dial-up networking is installed

- Click on the **My Computer** icon and see if a **Dial-up networking** box exists. If it does proceed to Step 2; if not follow these instructions (you will need to have your Windows95 installation disks to hand).
- Click on **Start I Settings I Control Panel I Add/Remove Programs I Windows Setup I Communications**
- Select **Dial-up Networking** and press **OK.** The appropriate files will be copied from the Windows95 CD-ROM or floppy disks.

Step 2 Install the Microsoft client

- Click on **Start I Settings I Control Panel I Network I Configuration I Add**

Table D.1 Typical TCP/IP settings

Requirement	Example	Role
Your own IP address	158.152.60.10	Identifies who you are
Your host name Domain name suffix	rkiley demon.co.uk	This combination is the text equivalent of the IP address
Provider's name server	158.152.1.65	Converts names into numeric IP addresses
Provider's default gateway	158.152.1.65	A gateway connects two networks that would otherwise be incompatible (here, your computer to your provider's network)
Provider's subnet mask	255.255.255.0	This number, combined with your IP address identifies which network your computer is on
Protocol you are using	PPP	Informs your provider which protocol you are using

- **Network Component Type | Client | Add**
- **Manufacturer | Microsoft | Client for Microsoft networks | OK**

Step 3 Install the TCP/IP protocol

- Click on **Start | Settings | Control Panel | Network | Configuration | Add**
- **Network Component Type | Protocol | Add**
- **Manufacturer | Microsoft | TCP/IP**

Step 4 Install the dial-up adaptor

- Click on **Start | Settings | Control Panel | Network | Configuration | Add**
- **Network Component Type | Dial-up Adaptor | Add**
- **Network Adaptors | Microsoft | Dial-up Adaptor**

Step 5 Configuring TCP/IP

- Click on **Start | Settings | Control Panel | Network | Configuration | TCP/IP | Properties**
- In the **IP Address Tab** complete your **IP address** and **Subnet mask**, as supplied by *your* Internet provider (Fig. D.1).
- On the **Gateway Tab** type in the **Gateway address**, as supplied by *your* Internet provider.

- On the **Bindings Tab** ensure that the **Client for Microsoft Networks** is checked.
- On the **DNS Configuration Tab** complete the **Host name**, **Domain name**, **DNS Search Server**, and **Domain suffix** as appropriate to you (Fig. D.2).
- Restart Windows95. This will allow all these changes to take effect.

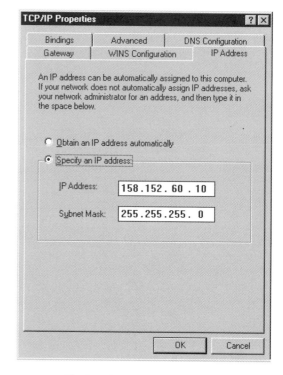

Fig. D.1 Defining the IP address

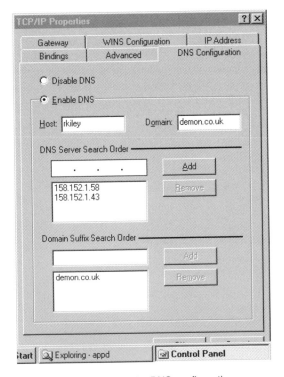

Fig. D.2 Defining the DNS configuration

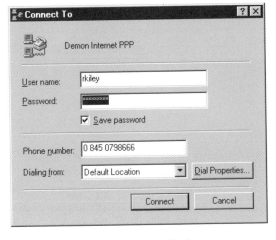

Fig. D.3 Connecting to the Internet

Step 6 Creating a dial-up connection to call your Internet provider

- Double-click on **Dial-up Networking** icon.
- Click on the **Make New Connection** and work through the 'New Connection Wizard' (that is, supply a name for this file – I called my file Internet – and the telephone number of your Internet provider).
- Click on the new Dial up icon, then select **File | Properties**
- In **Server Type** check that **PPP** is selected, (if you plan to use SLIP you will have to install this) and that the allowed protocol is **TCP/IP**

Step 7 Dial your provider

- Double-click your new dial-up icon.
- Enter your **User name** and **Password** in the appropriate boxes, and press **Connect** (Fig. D.3).
- Your modem will dial the number, and the settings you have defined will log you on to the Internet. When connected you will see a 'connected' screen similar to that shown in Figure D.4.
- Fire-up your Web browser, mail client, etc.

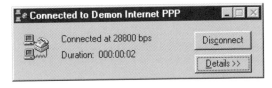

Fig. D.4 Connection acknowledgement

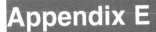

Glossary

applets *See* Java applet.

AT command language Language used by Hayes modems and equivalents. For example, to reset your modem you can type ATZ <carriage return>. For a complete set of commands see the documentation that came with your modem. As a rule of thumb most modems are supplied as 'Internet ready'.

BioMOO A virtual meeting place for Biologists (*see also* MOOs).

bookmark A way of 'recording' your favourite Web sites. Bookmarks negate the need to enter (or remember) long, complicated URLs. Bookmarks are the Netscape equivalent to Internet Explorer's Favourites.

bmp Bit mapped – a format for digitally storing an image. Alternative formats include gif and jpg.

bps Bits per second. A full page of text (in English) is approximately 16 000 bits. Thus a modem which can transmit data at 14 400 bps can send/receive the equivalent of just under one page of text per second (*see also* Kbps, Mbps and Gbps).

browser frames A way of helping users navigate through a complex Web site. Typically, two frames will be used: one frame will provide the contents page of the site and the other frame will display the specific link you wish to follow. As the 'contents page' is always visible, visitors to the Web site can quickly access another section without having to use the 'Back' button on the browser toolbar.

bulletin board system A computerised system which allows subscribers to post messages and exchange files.

cache A reserved space on a computer for storing items which are frequently requested. Your web browser, for example, caches pages from the World Wide Web to the hard disk. Thus when you want to go back to a previously accessed page your browser can retrieve it from the hard disk rather than from the original server.

client A computer program that requests the service of another computer, known as a server. Clients run on the local machine, processing and displaying information received from the server. For example, a World Wide Web browser is a client. For it to be able to do anything – display a page, etc. – it calls on the services of a Web server.

client software *See* client.

clock speed This refers to the speed at which the microprocessor – the 'chip' – in a computer can process information. This is measured in megahertz. The higher the number, the faster the computer will process data. Thus an advertisement for a 'Pentium 133' means that the computer has a Pentium 'chip' with a clock speed of 133 megahertz. A 'Pentium 266' computer is therefore faster (and more expensive).

CU-SeeMe An Internet video conferencing facility created by Cornell University.

CU-SeeMe reflectors If you wish to broadcast a conference using CU-SeeMe software you must route it through a CU-SeeMe reflector. Anyone who then wants to watch the broadcast can point their CU-SeeMe software at the reflector. If you are using CU-SeeMe on a *one-to-one* basis you do not route this through a reflector.

data compression To speed up data transfer most modems employ data compression facilities. The most popular of these are MNP5 and V42 bis. A modem equipped with V42 bis, for example, can multiply throughput by a factor of 4. Thus, in ideal conditions a 14 400 bps modem can receive data at speeds of 57 600 bps.

dial-up A dial-up connection uses phone lines to connect one computer to another via a modem. This is the easiest (and cheapest) way a 'home user' can connect to the Internet.

dialogue box Microsoft Windows applications use dialogue boxes as a way of communicating with you. Sometimes they may prompt you for information ('enter your search terms and press ok') and at other times they provide you with information.

DIP switches A set of switches which allow you to configure how your modem is set when it is first switched on (*see also* AT command language).

discussion lists Subject-specific discussion groups that are participated in and distributed by e-mail. Sometimes referred to as mailing lists.

domain name The unique address of a computer on the Internet. It comprises 'subdomains' that are used to group computers together. Thus all computers with **.uk** in their domain name are located in the UK. Those which are part of the academic community are identified by the name **.ac.uk,** whilst those computers located in commercial sites are assigned the name **.co.uk** (*see also* IP Address).

e-mail A medium for transferring information from one location to another. This can be in the form of a text or binary file.

e-mail address An e-mail address is made up of several parts. Thus the address abc@myplace.demon.co.uk consists of:

user name:	**abc**
host subdomain:	**myplace**
host name:	**demon**
type of organisation:	**co**
country:	**uk**

e-mail signature Text that is automatically appended to every e-mail message you send. Typically, this will consist of your name and contact address. Good netiquette dictates that this should never be more than three lines long, and that pictures drawn from text characters should be avoided.

Embase A pharmacological and biomedical database consisting of more than 7 million citations. The database focuses on the pharmacological effects of drugs and chemicals.

encoded When you attach a binary file (for example a wordprocessed document) to an e-mail message it is necessary to 'package' the attachment in a particular way so that the mail transport system can carry it. This is known as 'encoding' (*See also* MIME).

error correction A set of protocols used by modems to ensure that the data they receive matches that which was sent. If in any way the data is corrupted it will be retransmitted by the host server.

FAQ Frequently asked questions. Typically used to explain the purpose and function of a discussion list or newsgroup.

favourites A way of 'recording' your favourite Web sites. Favourites negate the need to enter (or remember) long, complicated URLs. Favourites are the equivalent to Netscape bookmarks.

finger A computer program that displays information about a user (or users) currently logged on to a local or remote system.

frame links Hypertext links contained within frames. A number of search engines experience difficulties indexing frame links.

freenets An organisation that provides free Internet access to its 'members'. Typically, freenets are established in public libraries, thus providing everyone with the opportunity to access the Internet.

freeware Software made available without charge.

FTP File transfer protocol. The most common method of moving files between Internet sites.

gif Graphics interchange format. A graphics file format used on the Internet.

Gopher A hierarchical menu-based system for exploring the Internet. Though this method of exploring has been completely superseded by the development of the World Wide Web, you will still encounter gopher-based resources on your trawls of the Internet. All resources stored on gopher servers can be accessed through a Web browser.

handshaking A term used to describe how modems regulate the flow of data between computers and modems to ensure data is not lost. For example, if data is transmitted more quickly than the computer can receive it, the handshaking process will send a message to the transmitter to wait. When the computer has processed that data and is ready for more, another message is sent requesting the transmission to recommence.

helper applications Helper applications extend your browser's abilities. For example, on its own Netscape *cannot* display video clips. If, however, you have a client which can play videos you can configure Netscape to launch this 'helper application' whenever a video appears on a Web page.

home page A starting point for Internet exploration.

host computer A host computer is one which *provides* interactive services – such as Telnet and FTP – to users on the Internet.

HTML A coding language used to create hypertext documents for use on the World Wide Web. For example, to indicate that a piece of text should be displayed in a bold font the term is prefixed with the code <B> and suffixed </b>. For help in authoring your own HTML pages see the collection of resources at:
**http://www.yahoo.co.uk/
Computers_and_Internet/
      Information_and_Documentation/
Data_Formats/HTML/**

HTTP Hypertext transfer protocol. The protocol for moving hypertext files across the Internet. Requires an HTTP client at one end and an HTTP server at the other.

hypertext A facility that allows related documents to be linked together. Selecting a hypertext link automatically displays the related document. Thus files held on different computers (in different parts of the world) can be linked together, providing a seamless integrated information resource.

image maps A Web graphic – usually a gif or jpg picture – composed of multiple (divided) regions, each linked to a URL. Image maps cut down on the amount of HTML code you have to write and stores all your links in one accessible location.

Internet Explorer A World Wide Web browser developed by Microsoft.

Internet provider A company or organisation that provide its clients with access to the Internet. For a fee, commercial providers allow individuals to connect their personal computers to those of the Internet provider; the provider's computers are permanently connected to the Internet.

Internet relay chat (IRC) A method of 'talking', that is, typing and reading messages in real time with groups of people via the Internet.

IP address Every computer on the Internet has an IP address, known colloquially as the 'dotted quad'. An example of an IP address is 158.152.1.65. Domain names are the plain language equivalents (*see also* Domain name).

Java applet A computer program that can be included on an HTML page. When you use a Java-compatible Web browser to view a page that contains a Java applet, the applet's code is transferred to your system and executed by your browser. The Java programming language was developed by Sun Microsystems Inc.

Java-compatible A browser capable of running Java applets.

JANET Joint Academic Network. The network which links all UK higher educational establishments.

JPEG Joint photographics expert group. A file format for images. JPEG files tend to be smaller than their 'gif' equivalents.

See JPEG.

kbps kilobits per second.

mailing lists *See* discussion lists.

MB Megabyte(s). 8 bits = 1 byte; 1 million bytes = 1 MB.

Mbps A million bits per second (*see also* bps, Kbps, Gbps).

MEDLINE Incorporating the printed *Index Medicus*, *International Nursing Index* and the *Index to Dental Literature*, MEDLINE is the largest biomedical bibliographic database. Dating back to 1966, MEDLINE has around 9 million citations drawn from around 3600 journals.

MeSH Medical subject headings. The thesaurus devised by the National Library of Medicine and used to index all articles in the MEDLINE database.

mirror To meet the demand placed on some FTP and Web sites, mirror sites were devised. As the name implies, these sites contain an exact replica of the original site. Netscape, for example, mirrors its FTP site to numerous locations throughout the world. To speed up data transfer 'local' mirror sites should always be used. All things being equal, users in the UK will find that it is quicker to FTP the Netscape browser from the mirror site at Imperial College than from the main Netscape FTP site in the US.

MIME Multipurpose Internet mail extension. A standard for attaching non-text files (such as wordprocessed documents, spreadsheets etc.) to e-mail messages. An e-mail client which can send and receive attached files is said to be 'MIME compliant'.

Modem MOdulator DEModulator. A piece of hardware that allows computers to communicate with each other through the telephone network.

MOOs Multiuser domain, object orientated. The accepted definition of a MOO is that 'it is an Internet accessible, text mediated virtual environment well suited for distance learning'. The easiest way to understand a MOO is to visualise it as a series of rooms, within which multiple individuals can congregate and interact. To move to another room you can type in cardinal directions, or if the MOO has a Web interface (like BioMOO), simply point and click to whichever room you wish to visit.

MPEG Moving picture expert group. A format for storing moving images (videos) (*see also* Quicktime).

multicasting Multicasting allows *one* user to send packets of data to *several users* for conferencing over the Internet. Video conferences delivered through CU-SeeMe use multicasting technology.

netiquette The etiquette of the Internet. The key element in netiquette is remembering that real people are on the other end of a computer connection.

Netscape A World Wide Web browser developed by Netscape Communication Corporation.

newsgroups A worldwide system for the electronic exchange of news and views on a particular topic. Also referred to as Usenet News.

newsreader Software which is used to read messages sent to Internet newsgroups. A good newsreader will sort the messages by the subject line so that replies are shown next to the original message.

NHSnet An Intranet established for the exclusive use of the National Health Service in the United Kingdom.

NLM UMLS National Library of Medicine Unified Medical Language System. A metathesaurus that provides a uniform, integrated distribution format from about 40 biomedical vocabularies and classifications and links many different names for the same concepts.

NNTP Network news transport protocol. The set of rules which dictates how Usenet News is propagated around the Internet.

NNTP server A computer (server) which you access to obtain Usenet News.

offline Not connected. In terms of the Internet this phrase is used to indicate that you are not connected, via the telephone line, to your Internet provider.

pdf Portable document format. Documents written in pdf can only be viewed if you have a pdf viewer, typically the Adobe Acrobat. A pdf file retains all the characteristics of a traditionally printed page – font, layout, pagination etc. – and it cannot be edited by the user.

PICS Platform-independent content selection. A method of rating Web pages, akin to the certificates awarded to motion pictures.

PING Packet Internet gopher. PING is used to test or time the response of an Internet connection. PING sends a request to an Internet host and waits for a reply. When you PING an address, you get a response telling you the number of seconds it took to make the connection.

platform dependent When you buy a piece of software – such as a wordprocessing package – you have to make sure that it is compatible with your operating system. IBM-compatible PCs run under DOS or Windows. Apple Macs run under the Macintosh operating system. In contrast, the Internet is *not* platform dependent. Any computer which has a copy of TCP/IP can connect to the Internet.

plug and play A term used by both hardware and software developers to describe their products. In essence it means that the product does not require any special configuring before it can be used. Open the box, plug it in and use it. Plug and play software will typically come with an 'installation' program, which will prompt you for any necessary information.

PoP Point of presence. Most Internet provider will create local points of presence to enable users to access the Internet through a local telephone number.

POP3 Post Office protocol, version 3. A set of rules designed to allow single users to read mail from a server. When e-mail is sent to you, it is stored on the server until accessed by you (*see also* SMTP).

point of presence *See* PoP

PPP Point-to-point protocol. A protocol that allows dial-up users to connect to the Internet and use TCP/IP-compliant clients. The alternative to PPP is SLIP.

processor size The microprocessor (or chip) is the main factor that determines how fast a computer can process data. A 386 chip is faster than a 286 but slower than a 486.

proxy server Rather than go directly to the server that hosts the data you require, you can instruct your Web browser to visit a 'proxy' server first. If the data you require is held on the proxy it will be delivered to your desktop more quickly than if it had to be fetched from the original host. If the data is not present on the proxy, then the Web browser will automatically request the data from the host server. If your Internet provider supports proxy servers I would recommend configuring your Web browser to access them (Appendix B).

public reflector *See* CU-SeeMe reflectors.

querybox An on-screen form through which you can input queries. An Internet search engine will have a query box where you can enter the subject you are searching for.

Quicktime A format for storing moving images (videos) developed by Apple (*see also* MPEG).

RAM Random access memory. An allocation of space where the computer *temporarily* places software applications and the operating system for high-speed access. The more you have, the faster your computer will work. 4 MB of RAM is the minimum required for Windows 3.1, whilst 16 MB of RAM is recommended for Windows95.

Real audio Software developed by RealNetworks for listening to sound clips over the Internet.

relevance feedback The process of using a document, retrieved from an initial search, to further refine your search. That is, once a relevant document has been found, you instruct erver to find 'more of the same'.

robots Computer programs which scour the Internet looking for new resources to index and check that previously identified sites are still available. Retrieved data is added to an Internet database. These databases can be interrogated using a search engine.

search engines A computer program which will undertake a search of an Internet database based on the information you have supplied.

server A computer that provides a service to client software running on other computers.

shielded modem cable The cable which connects the modem to the PC should be encased in braid or aluminium foil. This ensures that electrical frequencies from other appliances do not interfere with the data transmission process.

SLIP Serial line Internet protocol. A protocol for using a telephone line (a serial line) and a modem to connect a computer to the Internet (*see also* PPP and TCP/IP).

SMTP Simple mail transfer protocol. A protocol used to transfer e-mail between computers.

sound card A piece of hardware in the computer which allows the user to hear computerised audio clips via external speakers.

subject catalogues An Internet subject catalogue indexes the resources of the Internet into broad subject areas, in the fashion of a library.

SuperJANET The high-speed optical computer network developed for the academic community in the UK.

T1 Line A very fast data line, capable of transmitting/receiving 1 544 000 bits per second. In pages of A4 text this is equivalent to just under 100 pages per second.

TCP/IP Transmission control protocol /Internet protocol. Protocols which provide the basic transport mechanism for sending and receiving data on the Internet. Without TCP/IP you *cannot* connect to the Internet.

telemedicine The use of electronic means to deliver health care to persons at some distance from the provider.

Telnet An Internet service that allows your computer to directly connect and interact with a remote computer.

terminal adapter Hardware device used to connect a computer to an ISDN line.

uniform resource locator A way of specifying the Internet access method and location for any file/document held on the Internet. Locators consist of three parts. Thus the URL **http://www.who.ch/home.html** means:

http://	access method – in this case the hypertext transport protocol
www.who.ch/	the address of server
home.html	the directory path and file name, that is, where the file is on the server.

upload Just as one can download data from a Web site to a computer, it is possible to upload data to a Web site. Typically, this is done using FTP. Obviously, you can only upload data to sites to which you have been given full FTP rights, i.e. if your Internet provider gives you personal Web space on their server, privileges to add files to this site will be restricted to yourself.

URL *See* Uniform resource locator.

Usenet News *See* Newsgroups.

UNIX An operating system designed specifically to let many people access the same computer simultaneously.

V90 ITU standard A standard ratified by the International Telecommunications Union that ensures that all modems using this standard can 'talk' to each other at speeds of 56 K, no matter what company makes them or in what country they are used.

virtual reality A computer-generated simulation of a real environment. Thus, in a virtual reality environment the computer can generate visual, auditory or other sensual inputs, and the user can interact and directly manipulate objects within this virtual world.

viruses A virus is a computer program that can infect other computer programs by modifying them in such a way as to include a copy of itself. The term is used loosely to cover any sort of program that tries to hide its malicious function and tries to spread onto as many computers as possible.

waiting for host to respond A message displayed by the Web browser to indicate that the Internet server you are trying to contact is not responding. As a rule of thumb if you do not get a response within a minute it is best to sever the connection and try another time.

wizards Recognising that many computer-related tasks can be difficult, programmers have devised 'wizards' as a means of providing clear step-by-step instructions. Wizards range in complexity from the relatively simple – how do I insert a table in Microsoft Word – through to the complex, such as installing memory cards or connecting to the Internet.

WebTV A way of accessing Internet services such as World Wide Web and e-mail via your television set.

word spamming A method of deliberately repeating keywords on your Web page in an attempt to increase the likelihood that your site will be returned in the first few hits of a Web search. To determine the order in which matching documents are returned on the results page, most search engines use a ranking algorithm, based on the frequency with which the search term appears.

World Wide Web A global system that links information on the Internet through hypertext links embedded within documents. World Wide Web documents can contain graphics, moving images and sound.

World Wide Web browser Client software which can display any file that has been created using the hypertext markup language (HTML).

Index